My life as a miracle

a life of fighting cancer

Mar 19 2003

To my Good Friend RICHARD

Dominick J. Budnick

Dominick J Budnick

Printed in Victoria, Canada

National Library of Canada Cataloguing in Publication Data

Budnick, Dominick J., 1921-
    My life as a miracle : a life of fighting cancer / Dominick J. Budnick.

ISBN 1-55395-412-2

    I. Title.

RC265.6.B83A3 2002   362.1'96994'0092   C2003-900028-1

TRAFFORD

This book was published *on-demand* in cooperation with Trafford Publishing.
On-demand publishing is a unique process and service of making a book available for retail sale to the public taking advantage of on-demand manufacturing and Internet marketing. **On-demand publishing** includes promotions, retail sales, manufacturing, order fulfilment, accounting and collecting royalties on behalf of the author.

Suite 6E, 2333 Government St., Victoria, B.C. V8T 4P4, CANADA
Phone   250-383-6864   Toll-free 1-888-232-4444 (Canada & US)
Fax   250-383-6804   E-mail sales@trafford.com
Web site www.trafford.com   TRAFFORD PUBLISHING IS A DIVISION OF TRAFFORD HOLDINGS LTD.
Trafford Catalogue #02-1127   www.trafford.com/robots/02-1127.html

10   9   8   7   6   5   4   3   2

CONTENTS

My Life as A Miracle
Dominick Budnick

Date: April 1, 1990

Place: Bathroom, my house

Time: 3 a.m.

Writing my book dedication

To all my friends, doctors, relations, my children who in past years suggested I write a

book on my miraculous life.

I have had cancer most of my adult life it seems, and its been quite a fight to go on living

and continue on with this life of mine. My friends and family, if you think you are having a

tough time or are in pain and misery read this book. When you are done you will feel

much better and now how lucky and healthy you are,

Entrance:

My cancer surgeries started in 1949. Malignant cancer under left armpit, removed 1 year
later.

Malignant cancer under right armpit, then tumor cancer right breast., removed.

Cancer on top shoulder was removed=tumor with deep roots.

Cancer surgery, right temple then cancer tumor right eye, cancer left cheek opened up,
cancer removed.

1985 terminal cancer prostrate cancer all lower parts removed.

1990 cancer terminal tumors on organs.

1999 removed testicles.

2000 tumor back of head.

Stories of above in book.

Amen,

Dom

Chapter 1

Humble Beginnings

I was born in the year 1921 on July 2nd in Clatsop County in the foothills of Oregon's coast. I came into the world at 9 a.m. in the morning at St. Mary's Hospital. My father, Gus Budinich, was born on the island of Velli Losyin in the Adriatic Sea. He died in an accident at age 32.

My mother was born Katie Tarabochia on Woody Island in Washington State. She died in 1973. My family was originally Austrian. Grandma and Grandpa came from a small island in the Baltic Sea called Sonsego. That same island is now called Susak. At the time my grandparents were there it was, and still is, under Austrian rule.

I was baptized on July 10, 1921 at St. Mary's Star of Astoria. Our family was of the Catholic faith. My mother, Katie had five boys by the age of 25. My oldest brother's name was John and he died during the flu epidemic in 1919. My brother Joseph also died of the flu in 1919. He was 2 years old. My other brothers were Mike, he was 2 ½ years older than me and Gus who was named after my father.

The death of my father was hard on our family. He had been duck hunting when the accident happened. His friend Charlie Souderberg shot him by accident. I was born 7 months later.

At the time of my dad's death my mom went to Portland to the hospital. My dad's brother Marco and his family lived there. My mom was told that she could either have an abortion and not have me or live with the pregnancy. She could not read or write and she already had two small children and no way to support them. She had no money and no

where to go and many people told her it would be hard but she told me a story when I

was young about one night in the hospital. She said a catholic nun who was a nurse came

into her room and talked with her. She said the nurse was dressed completely in white.

My mother said that the nurse told her to have me and that made her decision. I was born.

My dad wanted me named Dominick if I was a boy.

My mother told me a few stories about my deceased brothers over the years. One story

bothered me a little but it seemed to help her to tell it.

It was 11 miles from our town of Brookfield Wash to a bigger town called Cathlamet. My

grandpa fished all night long and came home. Now consider this, you are a grandpa and

you have to take a grandchild of yours who had just died, and wrap him in a blanket. It

would be painful for anyone but that wasn't the end of the story. My grandpa took a loaf

of bread and a jug of wine and went to his boat carrying his grandchild. He put the child

in the boat and put him in the seat in the stern. He got into the boat too and silently

started rowing up the Columbia River against the tide. He rowed for hours and his big

powerful arms pulled the boat slowly up the river finally reaching the town of Cathlamet.

He picked up his grandchild and looked at him. What must have been going through his

mind as he looked at that little body wrapped in a blanket? His heart must have been

breaking. He picked up his grandchild and carried him the last mile to the little church

that, to this day, still stands on the side of the hill overlooking the great Columbia River.

St. Catherine was its name and it was built in the 1890's.

Grandpa finally got to the church and the Father of the Parrish took his grandchild and

put him in a small coffin. They said a few prayers over him and laid him in the ground to rest in peace. Grandpa then went back to the boat and rowed back down the river. He

rowed for approximately 34 hours up to Cathlamet and back. He rowed until he was tired.

He finally got home and to the door only to discover my grandmother and my mother

crying and pointing to my other older brother, his body wrapped in a blanket. He had died

during the night. His name was Joseph after his grandpa and he was only 2 1/2 years old.

Grandpa turned around and with little Joey in his arms and a little sack of food, went

back to his boat and again up the river, this time with his namesake Joey. He took Joey to

the little church and to the Father to be buried along side his brother. My mother said

Grandpa came home that night and slept 20 hours. My Grandma said to go through what

Grandpa went through must have been hard. It must have been hard looking at those

babies in the stern of the boat. How many people would have to take a valium or other

pills? How many doctors would we have to see and visit before we would forget a couple

of small boys who have gone on to rest in peace? I was told, however, that Grandpa woke

from his sleep and never said a word though his heart must have been breaking. He went

to the docks and worked on his nets and went out fishing as usual.

Grandpa worked hard until he was 79 years old. His heart gave up then and he passed

too. I remember the last time I saw my grandpa. He was sitting in his big chair and his

son's, My uncles Dominick and Joe carried him to the dock and he waved good-bye to us

all as the river boat took off down the river as his had done so many times in his life. I

never saw my grandpa again. The great man had left us forever.

I lived in a little town on the Columbia River called Brookfield. The town had no roads

out and was landlocked. It was a fishing town of about 300 people. There was a big

cannery for handling fish and approximately 25 fishing boats for the company owned by people named Meglar. Mr. Meglar ran the town which operated same as coal mines did.

Fishermen fished all seasons and the company took the fish in payment for a living in the

town. Fish paid for food, clothing and any thing else you needed. The company took

payment from the fish you caught. Most of the time people were way in debt to the

company and never caught up even on the books. Instead of being a coal miner's

daughter, I was a fisherman's son. It was the same thing though.

There was only one way in and one way out of town, by riverboat. The old paddle river

boats such as The America, the Norline and the Georginana were all big river boats. They

brought us our grocery order and mail every day. My mom used to make out a grocery

list and give it to the boat captain that came from Portland and went on to Astoria,

Oregon. The captain, who was Ernie Foster, and his brother ran the boat. They brought

the groceries that were ordered back and delivered them to the families on the way back

up the river. They were paid .25 cents for each order.

The boats that worked the river were the Julia B, the Molly B, The Imperial and one of

the boats that worked the river back then, The Virginia, is now up on Lake Washington.

It is used as a party boat in the Sound and Lake Washington.

Life was just plain. There was the fish cannery that had Japanese workers and a couple of

their families. There were also Chinese, a dozen or so, who only worked in the cannery

and lived in houses built on the water. There were about 200 of the people in town who

were related. There were cousins, uncles, aunts and etc. Most all the TaraBochia's, my

grandpa's people were there. My grandparents had four daughters and two sons. The

daughters, my aunts, were younger. My mom was the oldest. My aunt Zena married Mike

Scrivanich and they had four sons of their own and one girl. My aunt Donna married

Tony Churlin and they had six children. Uncle Tony was a big part of my life. (I'll

explain that further later in the story.) My aunt Nicholena married a logger or a mill

worker, I can't remember what position in the mill he held.

My mother had two brothers, Uncle Joe, who had 7 children and Uncle Dominick, who

had three boys and one girl. My cousins, who by the way had up to 11 children in one

family and 12 in another, were all around. All in all I have 1st cousins, 2nd cousins and 3rd

cousins and there is probably at least a 1000 of us if we were to have a family reunion.

Most of our families are commercial fisherman who have fished from California to the

Columbia River to Puget Sound to Alaska. We are all hard working, honest people.

Our little town produced many millionaires who left when the cannery burned down in

1929. People like the Zankich family who left for California and later went into the fish

cannery business eventually having one of the biggest fish market in California. Some of

the older folks bought lemon and orange farms in California and all became millionaires

that way. The Martinezes from Everett became top commercial fish captains, captains

and purse seine boat owners. They became tops in Alaska and Puget Sound. The Zorich

family moved to Seattle and became apartment owners, grocery store owners, fishermen

and in a family of 9 children, all became millionaires by the 1950's. 60's and 80's.

Tarabochia's, Scrivanich's, Bozanich, Suich and Churlin families also the Japanese

family of Tanaka moved to Seattle and became apartment building owners and millionaires.

Chapter 2

My Early Life

1921-1929 –

My life was just plain. We had a school house that was 100 yards from our house. We lived with grandpa and grandma in an old fish company house with a wood stove and oil lamps. There was no power, no lights and wood floors that were scrubbed on hands and knees with a brush. The house was unpainted and there was an out door toilet. There was running water but it came from the Jim Crow Mountain behind the town. The water flowed from a dam that was full of fresh mountain water. It was big enough that the cannery operated on the stream that ran through the mountains.

The school house was something else. It had two classrooms. First to fourth grade was in one room and fourth grade to eight grades was in the other. The teachers came fresh from college in Bellingham. They were good teachers and we learned to read, write, spell, math, geography and history. The teachers in the old days came to teach and the kids learned. We did as we were told and if we got out of line there was the switch but if we were good they rewarded us.

My teacher from the first grade was Violet Graham, a very nice teacher. She was only 21 years old and a very good teacher. She and her family lived in Bellingham. They had a small farm, about 8 acres.

Now the cannery burned down in Brookfield and my mother had no job. My brothers were too young and I was only 8 years old so my mom and grandma were left to support three little boys and themselves. We had a few chickens and a big garden but that was it.

Grandma and mom didn't know how to read and write which made it worse. Things were a lot harder for those who couldn't do either. Summer came and my mom shipped my brother Mike up to Portland to my dads' brothers' home. My uncle had nine children and was a fish peddler. He went door to door as a salesman peddling fish. He would take one of my brothers each summer. My school teacher took me. I spent my summers on her dads' farm in Bellingham. What an experience that was for a small country boy who had never seen cars and buses or even trains. (To this day I have still never ridden on a train.) My summer trips were like a whole new life. I was kind of lonesome and scared at first. I missed my mother and the family but that was how it had to be. It was the best for all of us, the only way to exist.

The Grahams were real nice people. Violet, my teacher, had an older sister whose name was May and we slept in the attic of their old house. I had a small bed by a window and it had a lot of spiders and flies in it. I remember being kind of afraid the first night or two but after a while they became friends of mine.

I was shocked the first morning when I was awakened about 5 a.m. and told to get dressed fast, Old Man Graham was waiting at the kitchen door for me with a couple of big baskets. He said my first job when I got up each morning was to go out to the chicken pen and get eggs. I picked out about 100 eggs each morning at 5 a.m., and then I washed up.

There was a big breakfast of eggs, bacon or ham and hot cakes each morning. After breakfast we would each get a hoe, the two girls, grandpa and me and go out to some acre long rows of carrots, beets, peas, beans and corn and hoe the weeds by hand till noon. A big bell would then ring and it was lunch time.

After lunch there was a siesta for an hour or so and then out to the fields again until about

3 p.m.

There was a nice big stream of water with a couple of pools. We would jump in and cool

off. The day would end with a big dinner and then early to bed. This was my life when I

was 8 years old.

My birthday was July 2 and I turned 9. It was 1929 and the Depression was in full swing.

I learned a lot in the years that followed. I was glad when I saw the big black taxi drive

up in the yard of the farm and I saw my mother get out and put her arms out for me. My

little heart broke and I cried.

My mom picked me up and took me to a different life. The cannery had burned down and

there was no work. There were not a lot of people were left in town. A few families, my

uncle Joe and my uncle Dominick, the Greget family, Harlou family and the Ashley

family were still in Brookfield. They fished and tenders picked up the fish they caught.

That's how they lived for a few years.

My uncle Tony and his wife Donna finally talked my mom into moving to Seattle and

living with them in a house on Barret Street, one block from the big city dump called

Interbay. This is where my life started all over again.

City life is much different from country living. There were cars for the first time and I

have to admit I was awful scared. It took me a while, at least a few weeks, to leave the

house and just go out. Fall had come though now and I had to start school which was

very different from the country school I was used to.

When I finally went we went to learn. We had to learn, my mom wanted us to, so I went

to St. Margaret's Catholic School and that's where I learned discipline. I was also taught the difference between right and wrong. We were taught, not only by the teachers but also by the switch strap across our behinds. Many times I had welts across my behind and my hands were pretty red and swollen.

One day I got home from school and had welts ¼ inch across the top of my legs and my behind. My brother Gus saw the welts and told my mom. She and my brother Gus took me back up to the school to Father Corboys house. I had to take my pants down in front of the Father and the Sister who had beaten me but when all the hollering had stopped they decided I had had it coming. My cousins, about 10 of us, got into the church before Mass on Sunday and went into the basement. A window was open and we climbed in and stole about 10 bottles of pop. The Father caught us. I learned then and there one of the important lessons for the rest of my life…don't steal. Many a time in my life I there after I could have stole different things but that beating stayed on my mind. I really had it coming that day. To this day I'm glad I got what I deserved.

The Sisters at the school were wonderful. They did all they could for us when they were teaching us. But back in those days we were considered a rough bunch of Slavs and the school was divided – the Irish kids against the Slav kids. I had about 20 cousins, all big guys, and we were always in some kind of trouble. Father Corboys would break a few hickory switches over our hands over the years. But as I said earlier I, or we, all got what was coming to us. Today that's what schools need; give the teachers the freedom to discipline children. That's why the world is like it is today. It starts with kids getting away with things at school. If they got punished for things they did wrong it would be a better place, but it is the teachers who get punished today.

We came to Seattle and lived with my uncle Tony. He had nine children of his own but

only six were living, three girls and three boys. These were my first cousins. Larry was

my favorite cousin and in later years we fished together on my boat and had great times

together. We were very close and I love him as if he were one of my brothers. Then there

were his brothers Anthony and Dewey as well as his sister Jean who was also like a sister

to me and finally, Catherine and Donna. All of them were hard workers and are still hard

working people today, except for Jean who passed away just last year of cancer.

They are all married and have nice families. They are doing fine today but back then we

all lived together and it was crowded. There were two families living in one small house

so for three or four of us to share one big old bed it was just living the best way we could.

All together there were 13 of us living at the house and the Great Depression was in full

swing. Boy was it a hard way to live. You can imagine having hardly any money, food

and clothes. But we all did the best we could.

Uncle Tony was a captain on fishing boats we call purse seiner. He was a captain on a

herring seiner in Alaska as well as fished for sardines in California He was gone nine

months of the year fishing. My brother Gus went with him for several years and he was

gone 6 months at a time. In 1930 Gus came home from Alaska and we moved to our own

little house across from the *on the* city dump. It cost us five dollars a month rent but we were on

our own.

We were so poor we used to get a lot of vegetables from the dump. Every Wednesday

and Saturday evening at 6:30 p.m. the old model A trucks would come from the public

market. There were also street peddlers who used to go down the street hollering "fresh

vegetables" who would come out and buy off the truck. There were also fish trucks. We would be on the dump, my mom and me. And they would fill a wash tub with the old vegetables, old lettuce, bananas and such. We would fill our tub and pack it up to the house. Ma would cut the bad parts out of the bananas, tomatoes lettuce and whatever else we could pick up. We had vegetables for the entire week that way. I remember the day my cousins and I were waiting for the trucks to come and a big ice cream truck full of quarts and pints of ice cream came a long. Something small was wrong with the ice cream so we loaded our tubs and brought it home. We had ice cream for a couple of days. We didn't have an ice box or a refrigerator; we only had a wood stove and a wood stove heater. We were, after all, a very poor family, but there were a lot of families in those days that were just like us.

My brother Gus was on the WPA and making $1 a day working. Mike and I were still too young to work, I was only 10 years old, but we did get some help from the church and St Vincent De Paul. They gave us a sack of flour a month and I got my first pair of long pants and some black and white shoes. I was in heaven, I was the only boy in school up to that time who wore sneakers up to my knees and I had hated them. I also had old shoes full of holes so the stuff the church gave me was great. I was one happy kid.

My mom got a job at the pickle factory and she walked for several miles every morning in second hand shoes through snow, cold and rain to get to work. She walked at least two miles or more to get to work and back. All that walking ruined her feet and toes in later years. They had to be operated on and cut under each toe. It was from having shoes that didn't fit, either too small or too big. She worked for $2 a day to feed us kids while grandma took care of the house.

I remember many a night when Ma and grandma were up until 12 midnight baking bread and washing clothes by hand. They would then go to bed and get up again the next morning at 6 a.m. so Ma could walk to work. That was hard and she really suffered.

The next few years from the age of 9 to 13, my life was mostly school, religion, First Communion at the church and conformation. It was a struggle, really, just to exist.

My summers were cutting lawns. We lived in the inner bay and I had a few friends of my own but I had to try and work. There were people who tried to help us by letting us cut their lawns. I would walk, bum a ride or thumb it all the way out to 100th and Greenwood where I had two customers whose lawns I cut. They were big lawns too and sometimes it took e up to four hours. They had to be trimmed and cut perfectly. I would work and sweat and then thumb my way back home. I got paid .50 cents and my mom would want the money right way so I cut more lawns for .75 or .50 cents a lawn all summer long.

I cried many times cutting those lawns, because I thought that these people were taking advantage of me, making me do all that work for .50 cents. But I cried myself out and continued to do it even though it was hard work. If I had only known what was ahead for me, I would have probably would have stopped.

At 13 years old I was too young to work a regular job so I was sent to my old hometown of Brookfield where I would spend the rest of my summer. I would stay with my uncle Joe and Aunt Winnie. They were really nice.

My mom put me on a bus from Seattle to Kalamawn, six hours away. This was where my uncle Tony, the one married to my mother's sister Nickolena, lived. She was my mothers' youngest sister. When I was sent there my aunt had already died two years earlier. Uncle Tony met me and took me to his home until 11 p.m. when we went down to the river docks where the old paddle wheel The America was running. We hung a

lantern out on a post and that was the sign for the boat to stop. At midnight I got aboard

for .50 cents and started on my way on the river. I lay on an old seat bench and listened to

the sounds. I heard the old squeaking of the old paddle wheel and old chairs and benches.

I listened until I feel asleep. Later I was put out on the dock in Brookfield.

I arrived at 4 a.m. at the break of dawn. I was afraid to awaken my uncle and his family

so I just walked around the old town. It was like a ghost town then. There were just two

families who permanently lived there and a couple of old time fishermen, Paulo

Marinkovich and his brother Anthony. They would come down from Portland during

fishing season.

John Asheley still lived back on a farm. Anton Fadich still lived in town for the few

summer months. There was also old Con Harlou, one of the oldest and smartest men I

ever knew. His family was the only real educated family who lived on the Jim Crow

creek. They lived about two miles back. There was also old Jack Ben and his wife who

lived in the woods with the bears and deer. They got to be over 100 years old. They came

into town one time a month and met the river boat, picked up a sack of flour and headed

back up into the woods. There's quite a history of those people in the early books written

on the history of the lower Columbia River. I could tell you a lot of stories too though.

At daylight I got to my uncles and the family was glad to see me. The house was live ours

with wood floors and all. I slept up in the attic with a couple of big wood rats who kind of

kept me awake packing stuff in-between the beams and all. I complained to my uncle one

evening and we heard them in the ceiling dragging things again. They usually drag in

leaves, branches anything they can get in the rafters. My uncle got out his shotgun, a 12 gage, and we got them lined up. He just shot three fast shots into the ceiling and a few

drops of blood came through. We knew out problem was over.

There were also bats that came in at night through holes and open vents. I lived with

those, we got along okay.

My fishing career started when I was 13 going on 14. I was at my uncles in Brookfield

for the who*le* summer and we went to Astoria to get his company boat from an old cannery

called Anderson's Fish Company. While there the cannery gave me a 26 foot old little

boat. It had a four horse power standard engine in it. They also gave me a floater net. It

was an old 100 fathom net and I fished with it on the beach in front of Brookfield. There

was an old quarry used for crushing rocks and I fished from there on to the old dock off

our town. It was quite an experience for a guy 13 years old. It was June and I would be 14

on July 2nd. I caught a few big salmon. One I remember weighed 54 ½ pounds. Boy was

he *b*ig. I stayed with Uncle Joe all summer that year. I made $191 for the whole summer

but at 13 years old that isn't too bad. The company takes 50 percent for the boat and gear

rental so I came home in the fall to attend the 8th grade and bought my first new pants,

shirt ad shoes. For the first time they weren't hand me downs or my brothers or from St.

Vincent De Paul.

I finally had made it to the 8th grade. It went fine. My grades were never too good and all

through my school career I was considered a dreamer. I would sit most of the school day

and look out the window of the school. I never did my homework so I was a C student.

Most of my report cards went something like, A- A+ - B – B+ - C – C+. I did my

spelling, reading, writing and arithmetic, that's how I got by in my eighth grade year. I

graduated from the 8th grade that was something else.

We were poor kids. A lot of people these days don't know what poor is. They have

welfare food stamps and all kinds of ways to get help now days but back then we didn't

have that. My mom didn't know how to read and write or even where to go for help

except for the Father at church. Ma got around a lot even though she could read. If she

wanted to ride the bus she would walk around until she found someone she could tell that

she had left her glasses at home and ask them if they would read the schedule and tell her

when a certain bus would come. She got all over the place by herself and by being wise.

She worked as a housemaid for several people, doctors and business people who had big

beautiful homes. She cleaned many a toilet in her life. She spent her days working,

washing and cooking, sometimes for just $1 or $2 a day. And when my mom cleaned a

home it shined. You could eat off the floors anytime. I remember when I was home many

times she would call and she had to open a can of fruit or vegetables but couldn't read the

cans. She would call the letters off to me one and a time over the phone and I would tell

her what it spelled. That was really hard for her. Now days most cans have pictures on

them that are easy to see. She could write or print her name though. And you could read it

when she did. That was it though. My mom was one of the hardest working women I

have ever seen and I loved her. I work like her now.

My high school years were something else. First I had to go to Queen Anne High. I had

to walk all the way up the hills for miles. The canal split the school zones so we could not

go to Ballard High just across the Ballard Bridge. It wasn't like it is today, buses and all.

Kids today have it easy. I would have holes in my shoes.

I remember the day Ma was so mad that I came home from school with holes in my

socks. She was so made she chased me around the house saying that I was dumb and didn't know any better. She said, you put cardboard in your shoes and take your socks off

and put them in your pocket when you leave from school. She said this would save my

socks and so that's what I did until we got shoes for me from St Vincent De Paul. That's

why my school books were always so thin, I used to tear three to four sheets out and fold

them up to put in my shoes till I got home. That was just the beginning of high school.

I had three cousins who went to school with me so we hung around together.

My brother Mike was a big star in high school. He was a baseball pitcher for the school

and one of the best. No one knew we were brothers. I was warned a few times by Mike

not to foul up his name in school. He would walk down the hall with girls on his arms

and I would sneak along the wall of the hall so I wouldn't interfere with the star of Queen

Anne High.

As days went by, things got worse. Winter for us, walking as we did, was hard. I would

skip school every other day. I would go with my cousins and we would get a dime

however we could and use it to bum to town. There was a theater in town called The

Green Parrot Theater on 1st and Pike. We would go every other day. They had a serial

running, The Last of the Mohicans. We used to, or I rather I would, write notes and sign

my mothers name. Or sometimes she used to sign and ask me what it said and I would

read the note as, "Dom is doing real good in school" or I would read whatever came into

my mind and Ma would sign it. I would then take the note to school and I was out, no

problem. I would say I had to go to the dentist or some good excuse as to why I couldn't

be in school.

I would go to class sometimes with terrible breath. I would have had an onion sandwich

from home because that's all we had, and my class after lunch, math, had a girl named

Violet Begis in it. I like Violet but she didn't even notice me except for my onion breath.

She smelled that and suddenly she noticed me for the wrong reason. I was really ashamed

and so I missed a lot of classes such as math. I was ashamed because I was poor.

In the spring my cousins and I went to school one day and all got slips to report to Mr.

Luther the school principal. We all ended up sitting in front of the principal's office and

he called my cousins in one and a time. They all ended up expelled from school. I was the

last one to walk in to the office and he told me to sit down. Mr. Luther started telling me

about my brother Mike and how good a student he was, how he got good grades and he

was good in sports. He said all he wanted to know was what had happened to me. Just as

I was about to answer my brother came into the office. Mr. Luther had sent for him. He

asked what did he do now and Mr. Luther explained that I had missed fifteen out of thirty

school days and that he had a hand full of notes from my mother. Mike was pretty mad.

He told Mr. Luther that my mom didn't know how to read and that the notes were all

forged. Mr. Luther asked Mike what he should do with me and Mike stuck his thumb out

and said, boot em out and that's exactly what happened. The principal said "Dom there's

nothing I can do but expel you from school. So I thanked him and ended up outside with

my cousins. We all went home.

Mike and I were good friends most of the time but I did take a few lickings from him.

That had no bearing on me leaving school though. So I ended up on my own. My mom

was pretty mad. My older brother was in Alaska at that time and I now had to get out of

the house. I wasn't put out by my mom but I now had to manage a life of my own. So

that was the end to my short high school career. I started out in high school as a freshman

and that's where it ended, as a freshman.

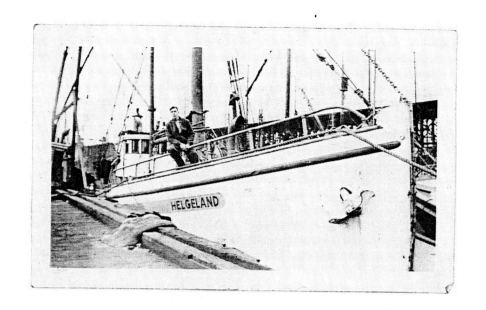

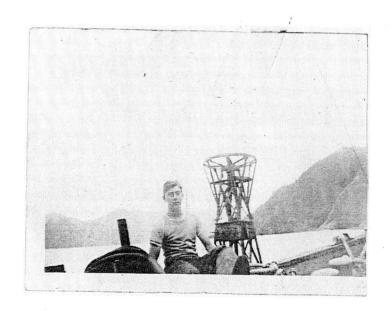

Chapter 3
Stowaway

At 14 years old and after just having been expelled from high school I wasn't sure what to

do next. My brother was mad at me. My grandma and my mom had just reddened my

bottom so I left and went down to hang out at the fisherman's terminal. I decided to leave

home.

After a short time I got friendly with a nice cook aboard a big halibut schooner tied up to

the dock. The schooner was The Helgeland and Captain Humes was a nice skipper. He

had a crew of 11 men. In later years, when the war broke out in 1941 the Helgeland went

north for Halibut season and never returned. The skippers' wife asked the Marshall's office

in Washington DC to check on the records of Japanese submarines and found out through

DC that the Helgeland had been used for target practice by the enemy subs. The schooner

was sunk, crew and all. They had been a real fine bunch of guys. It wasn't just service

men who lost their lives during that war.

Before all that though, I talked to the cook while the schooner was in dock for a few days

and ended up aboard it. I learned that they were going to leave so I kind of looked the boat

and spotted me a good place to hide. I went home soon after and got me a little bag and

threw a few things in it. I threw in some old clothes and an old torn coat I had and at 3:30

a.m. the next morning I was down on the docks sneaking aboard the boat. I hid in a rope

oar locker. I just squeezed in and stowed away. I ended up falling asleep and next thing I

heard was the engine running. I knew I had to stay hidden for quite a while or they might

turn back and dump me off. So I hid and cried for a while finally falling asleep again. After about 15 hours the door opened up and there stood the old cook. He

turned white as though I was a ghost. He grabbed me out and took me up on deck to the

skipper. Captain Hume and the crew were shocked but they said they would take me to

Ketchikan, Alaska. The crew then got together and each one gave me $1 so I could go to

a hotel in town when we got there.

The crew told me that once we got there to hang around the docks during the daytime and

watch for the Alaska steamships. The boats that were running at the time were the Old

Columbia, Baraoff, the Alaska and Denali. I was told to watch for one of these ships.

They told me to sneak aboard around midnight or later and go to the aft steering

compartment and hide behind the aft steering machine. When it started working, they

said, come out and I would be on my way back home.

They dropped me off on the dock in Ketchican and headed west and there I was 14 years

old standing on the docks in Alaska. My new friends were leaving me there alone so with

tears running down my cheeks, frightened I sat down on an old overturned big skiff.

What should I do, I thought? Where do I go from here? I pulled myself together and I

planned my next move. I was scared and I had $14 in my pocket. I didn't know anyone so

I decided to stay right on the dock so I wouldn't miss the ship that the crew had told me

would come. I put my sack of clothes under the big skiff and walked up town to the

grocery store. I bought me one bottle of strawberry jam, one jar of peanut butter, one

large loaf of bread and one quart of milk. I went back to my hideout on the dock and hid

all the groceries like a squirrel. I then started my watch for my ship. For the next few

days I walked around town and went up behind the town on a hill. There I ate a few

berries and looked on the channel watching for a ship that would take me home to my mom. After two days and nights of sleeping under that old boat, I slept on the seat on just

a plain old board and I was cold, I cried myself to sleep.

Finally, just as my friends from the schooner had promised when they put me off on the

dock, the Alaska steamship Columbia landed on the dock. I was about two miles up in the

woods when I heard this big whistle blow. Boy did I run for a clearing and there she was,

tied up to the dock. I ran all the way back to the docks and when I got there the dock was

loaded with people. There were so many people and work all going on at the same time

that I could not see anything. At first I couldn't see a way that I was going to get on that

ship so I stayed right there and watched for my chance. I had to stay up until 2 a.m. but I

finally got my chance to get aboard. There was no one around so I got my little bag and

climbed the gang way. I went to the stern and my heart was pounding so hard I thought

my ears would pop. I found this small hatch and steps and then the steam engine. I hid

behind it and it was nice and warm. I fell asleep and I felt good to be on my way home.

I was rudely awakened some time later by the big steam engine grinding and working. It

so happened that I was hid behind the big steam steering engine so the big propeller was

churning and it was loud. I came out and a Filipino fellow saw me. He took me up to the

bridge and I told him what I had done. He was very worried because he said this ship was

actually headed north, not back to Seattle. It was going to Prince William Sound. He

didn't know what to do with me now. I got a bunk with the Filipinos in the aft galley and

I had to wash dishes and set tables. I had to stay down with the stewards.

I got to see Juneau seaward and then after three days we arrived in Prince William Sound

to a cannery called Port Ashton. There the Captain said he had to drop me off because of

being afraid of a young kid getting hurt on the ship. Also the unions were active at that

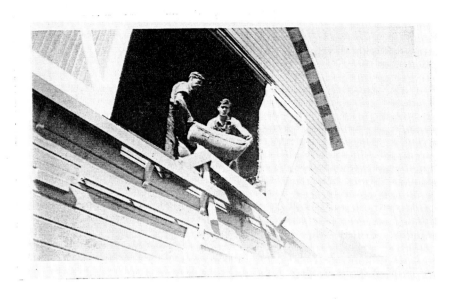

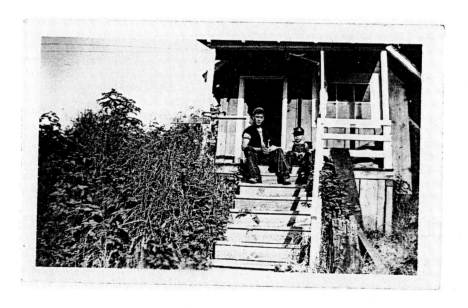

time and it was not considered right to have a young kid on the ship. So there I was on

the dock, no job, no where to go and I was crying and scared. I was standing with my

head down when a native fellow named Henry Morris heard my story and told me that a

herring plant called Hemlock Packing Company needed a man to work. I went to the old

cannery and who should I have a run in with but my Uncle Tony and my brother Gus.

They were real surprised to see me. They couldn't believe how I had gotten north. I

started working for the cannery as a fish feeder and for a kid 14 years old, doing this, a

man's job was great. I had already learned some hard lessons and had some hard times on

this voyage I took but what I didn't know was that the worse was yet to come.

A feeder job is opening a door with a handle that was on a gear when the fish, herring,

was unloaded from seiners into a huge round tank. They were as big as one small house

so I worked 12 hour shifts and then eat and sleep for 12 hours. It was long hours but good

food and a lot of sleep. It was tough working those shifts. The herring tanks were slanted

down toward the 3 foot by 3 foot door I opened. Herring spilled out into a worm type

deal that took the fish into being made into fillets and oil.

The oil is used for 70 different things but mainly soap of all different types. Now the job I

had was okay until the herring got to the bottom of the tanks and I ad to go into the big

tank with boots, oil skins and a big flat shovel. I had to push the fish through the hole. I

had to keep the fish coming through or I was in trouble. That fish used to stick like a

glove to the bottom of the tank and I would pull my guts out. I would cry trying to keep

the fish going in and boy I cried many a night also with my back aching my arms feeling

like they were falling off. I did it though and I did it all for $100 per month. That was the

pay I got and we would work for six months straight, a ship would come every month and pick up the herring that was bailed in sacks as well as a few thousand gallons of oil. The

boss William Hemlock would go down with the ships and collect the money for the

cargo. He would then put it in the bank and come up to get more. So the season went on

into the fall ad the wind and rain came but we worked on.

I had some times off and would go hunting. I used to hunt tumigan, something like a

grouse or at least it was part of the pheasant family. I got up to 22 in one or two hours. I

also got a few big eagles at that time eagles claws hanging on or nailed to your porch was

a nice trophy. There were also those big wings which could be as long as 6 feet, the

longer the prettier. The season was coming to an end and I was glad because it was long

and hard. I had turned 15 years old in July of that year so I was getting to be an old man

quickly. I worked with the older men up in the cannery, some guys in their late 20's and

30's. That was old for a kid like me then. The worst shock was yet to come though. I had

about $700 coming to me for my six months of hard labor but what we didn't know was

that the owner of the company William Hemlock took all the money that he got from the

oil and all, sold his home and ran off into Canada with it all. So we all went home.

I got to come home with my brother Gus and Uncle Tony. We had the Betty Jane which

was a solid 68 foot seiner. It had an old bolinde engine in it and as we left Prince William

Sound and started across the Gulf of Alaska, it is about a 32 hour run, we got caught in

one of the worse storms I've ever been in all my life. In all the years I was at sea that is

still the worse one I've ever been in. It took us 105 hours to cross that gulf. My uncle

who was 30 years old at the time was on the wheel most of the time. We lost everything

we had on the deck, it was completely cleaned off. I was so seasick that I didn't care if

we sunk or not. I had never gotten seasick and I haven't been seasick since then. We had a very good fisherman, Matt Nicholich on board. He had been fishing with Uncle Tony

and Gus but during that storm he threw on his cloth boots and oilskin over board and

never went back to sea or fished again after that trip. When we finally got to Seattle there

was no money for anyone so we put a lien against the cannery. (Today that cannery is just

dust. The last time I visited I noticed it had fallen.) I was home and safe though. My ma

and grandma hugged and kissed me. The runaway boy was home again. That was the

summer of 1937 and what followed was a real tough winter. There was no money so I got

a job working for some friends of my mom's. Mr. Joe Vccilini had a grocery store down

on Cedar Street five city blocks north of the main part of downtown. It was near Pikes

Street market and I used to bum a ride every day from Interbay to Cedar street, about ten

miles from home to get to the store first thing in the morning. I worked stacking the

shelves with food for two hours and then I would dust and sweep for an hour a day. I

would get a sandwich and a glass of milk, that was lunch, and then I would get a couple

of dollars and walk to the public market five blocks away and buy a crate of fresh

tomatoes or sometimes 2 crates packing one under one arm and one under the other. I

would walk back another five blocks to the store and start cutting firewood in the

basement of the old building until I had a cord of wood, stacking it by hand for 2 hours

each day. I would then get my pay of .50 cents and bum back home to Interbay. I did that

most of the winter. Ma would work for the Legaz family and make her $2 a day cleaning

house and toilets all day. Between the two of us we brought home $2.50. My brother Gus

worked for the W.P.A. for $1 a day that made $3.50. My brother Mike was finishing

school and he had his sports. He had a paper route on Pier or Garfield Street and 15th

Avenue. He kept his money though and used it for lunch and school supplies. We paid $5 a month for rent, bread was .5 cents a loaf, milk was .5 cents and hamburger was .10

cents a lb. Gasoline for a car was .15 -.16 cents a gallon but we didn't have one so that

was no big deal. We did have to buy wood though and that was $2-$3 a cord and I would

have to chop kindling every day for the stove and bring in wood up to the old wood box.

It was not an easy winter. It was cold but Mike and Gus and me all slept in the same bed

and sometimes I was in the middle so it would be warm. The bed had an old mattress and

springs and we all sunk into the middle where there was a big hole. I had slept with my

mom until I was 13 and then my brothers. But my grandma had her own bed. She was

sort of the head of the house. My brother Gus was a dad to us all. He was the oldest and

the job really had fallen to him. He was father to us all after my dad was gone. He took

over the family. That year I was 15, Mike was 17 and Gus was five years older than Mike

which made him 22 in 1939.

The winter passed and I was glad. We had Christmas every year and we got a pair of

socks, a small bag of candy, an orange, an apple and always some nuts. Usually somehow

ma would get a small turkey or ham for Christmas dinner. That happened for most of our

Christmas's. They were all very much the same; I don't remember ever getting a toy. In

fact, I don't remember ever getting a toy for my birthday or Christmas or ay other time

for that matter. I had no toys when I was small. I had my first birthday party in 1980

when I was 59 years old and my kids gave it to me. It was very special.

The spring of 1938 came and my brother Mike went off to play ball. Gus was going to

Alaska to fish with Uncle Tony and I was left at home. I wasn't there for long though. I

went begging for a job in the canneries in Alaska and with a little fibbing about my age, I

got a job in one of the canneries in Port Ashton, Alaska. I was a fertilizer sacker for $100 a month. I went on the old steamer Alaska and I arrived at the cannery in Port Ashton. It

was a big herring plant and salmon cannery. My uncle Tony's boat was there tied up to

the dock. They were sleeping because you fish for herring at night. I went aboard and

went down into the bow of the boat. The boat was the Fairfax and it was 68 feet with 6

men sleeping in the bow in bunks. Captain Uncle Tony and the cook slept in the captain's

quarters on deck. I went into the bow and there was my brother Gus sleeping. I tapped

him on the shoulder and he opened his eyes and looked at me. He said he thought he was

dreaming so he rolled over and went back to sleep. I tapped him again and he looked

back and realized it was me and jumped up. He said where the hell did you come from?

He got up and went on deck and I told my story. He was surprised.

We went up to the cannery and he introduced me to the bosses. After that I got my own

little cabin with a bed in it and an outdoor toilet. It was a real nice little cabin. There were

at least twenty of these little cabins with two of us in each one. My roommate was a

young guy named Harry Lane. He was a nice guy and he showed me all over the plant.

There was a nice mess hall and after walking around I was ready to go to work the next

morning.

The next day after a breakfast of eggs, bacon, hotcakes and milk, (I was in heaven with

that kind of food) I was named a meal sacker. When the fish was pressed and all the oil

was out of it, it went into big oval drums and heated. It then became dried chunks of

fertilizer and out through pipes. I had sacks piled up by the hundreds and I would open

them up, put them under the end of the pipe and step on a lever filling the sacks. I then

took the sacks out, sew them up with a big needle and thread and pile them up for the

truck to pick up.

This was another job that included 12 hour work days and it was hard. I was 15 years old

still because my birthday wasn't for another two months but I did my job. I worked for

several months when my cousin came to the cannery and said one of their crew members

got hurt. They wanted me to go fishing with them on the boat "Mars". The boat was

owned by Martin Budnick and his sons Sam and Elmer. They were all on board and

Martin Suich was running things as captain.

Herring fishing was one of the best parts of my life. It was real interesting and exciting.

We also had fun. I was with my friends about the boat. We had a cook named One-eyed

Pete and we all lived, slept and ate like one big family.

I remember the first night out fishing. We got a full deck load of fish. There was fish

from the bow all the way back, we were loaded down. There was even a chimney in the

galley for the stove and hen One-eyed Pete opened the top to light the stove herring fell

out. Boy was he surprised. The pipe opened up on the deck so as we had shoveled the

herring onto the deck we had also loaded up his stove with live fish. We had a cold

dinner that night.

The season went on and after 6 months we headed home to the south. That was a trip I

always dreaded. It was always the last of October and going into winter. The weather was

changing for the worse and we almost always had a storm trip home. On that trip we hit

one o the biggest breakers I've ever seen in all my years of fishing. The old Mars went up

on its side about 40 feet in the air and there was nothing below us. We came down on our

side and it knocked the cook and engineer out of their bunks. They both ended up with

broken ribs. All the seams opened up on our hull so we had to go in at a cannery called

Tennakee and we re-corked the hull and repaired all we had to. After that we started out for home again and arrived back at fisherman's wharf shortly after that. It had been a good season and I made $800 for the 6 months. My mom and grandma were glad to see me as usual; after all I was the baby in our family. Over the years I have heard that more than once. In fact I heard that every time we met someone. My mom would say, "This is my baby". Oh boy, I heard that for years.

After we got home I went fall fishing on a purse seine boat in the Puget Sound. The boat was the Silverland run by Captain Tony Martinez of Everett. He was one of the top fishermen on the Sound.

I was 15 years old and getting a little reputation of being a fisherman so I got the skiff man job which was a tough job on the boat at that time. For this job you were in a small skiff about 20 feet long with a net called a lead. The Seine boat goes up to the beach towing the skiff behind close as possible. The big seine would get into the shallow water then the skipper would turn the seine boat around and holler let go the lead. I would throw the end of the small net over board and the big boat would start out from the beach laying the net out behind it. After about 100 fathoms the skipper would holler let go of the net and those on the main seine, which was attached to the bow of the skiff, would pull a pin on the big net and it would come off the boat and lay out in a half moon circle. The big boat would then tow the big net for about 40 minutes or longer into a complete circle until it came back to my skiff. I would then throw up a line from my end of the big net and release the net to the big boat. I would then run to the stern of my skiff and have to pull the small net in. After a good back workout and sweating a lot I'd get the net in and the take the big oars out and start rowing back to the seine boat. Sometimes it would take at least two or three blocks away and that was back breaking work. Rowing that big skiff with heavy winds blowing against you made it harder. Sometimes the sea was rough and you had to get back as soon as possible because you had to start pulling corks on the bow of the big boat. Sometimes you ran and jumped up to the stern of the seine pulling corks there until your back ached. You would then start pulling in the big net by hand over a roller on the turn. The net set on the roller and when it was about all in you would get out the brailer, as we called it, and dip the fish caught and dump them into the big hatch. After the fish were onboard you would pull up the rest of the net quickly getting it and the skiff ready to do it all over again. I can tell you that about five or six sets or more a day and your bones and back were aching pretty badly. You really hit the bunk at night and before you even lay down you're asleep only to get up at sun up and do it all again the next day. We fished five days a week in those days.

I had one experience that fall that I remember well. My friend Henry Zuvich and I were fishing together. Henry and I have been friends for 60 years. He was quite a character, in fact I could write a whole book on Henry himself. We went through grade school together and the little bit of high school I attended. He was one of the boys I got expelled with.

Anyway Henry and I were fishing together that fall and we had fished several different seasons together on the Silverland. He was an engineer. We came in and had gotten aboard the boat in the Everett marina about 3 a.m. and at about 5 a.m. the other crew members came aboard. They were coming from their homes and everyone was ready for some good fishing. As the skipper went to start the engine it wouldn't start. It was out of air and the skipper was mad. There was some screaming and yelling and hell-raising before we finally turned out the bunk and got the auxiliary engine started to pump air into the big tank so we could get the 100 pounds of air needed into the bigger engine in order

to start it. The whole fleet had left and there we sat broken down. Competition in those

days was tough from day to day. It was also the end of the season so we needed to be on

our way.

There was heavy fog that morning and we were over an hour late getting started but when

we finally headed out we ran into a big school of silvers just a short distance out. They

were jumping all around us but the bay was closed to fishing or at least that area was. The

skipper decided thought hat because we had heavy fog we would try fishing it anyway.

He said we had to be real quiet and work as fast as we could. He said we could take a

chance on not getting caught and arrested. We made a set right there and picked up 1900

silver salmon and headed out to Bush point where we usually fished with the rest of the

fleet. We ended up the high catch boat that day.

The fall season ended and I came back to a big job. I went to work that winter for the

N.Y.A., the National Youth Administration, I walked from Interbay up to Fort Lawton

every day and worked as a carpenter's helper.

We built the barracks up at Fort Lawton. I worked hard eight hours a day on one

sandwich from home and water to drink. I made $16 a month on that government job.

That came to about .51 cents a day working in the cold and snow. Today there are jobs all

over town that go for $5 -$6 an hour, that's $50 a day and nobody will work for that.

That's the difference in the world today, the government gives out food stamps and

money if you are on welfare. You get more there than if you work sometimes. I can't

believe the world today. To learn to live and live reasonable we need a good solid depression to teach people how to live on $5 and not on government taxes paid by people

who work and all.

In 1939 my brother Gus was going fishing again with my Uncle Tony on the boat

Excellent. Tony Scrivnich was also with him that year and they had the same old crew.

My brother Mike was getting to be a celebrity in those days. He was a star baseball

pitcher for the Seattle Rainers in the Pacific Coast League and he was really good. We

used to go and watch him play at the old stadium in Rainer Valley. He was going up the

ladder quickly. He went to the big leagues up to the New York Giants. He got married

and moved to New York after that. He did real well up until the time the war came along

in 1941 and then he got drafted into the Navy. He ended up on a special baseball team

with the Navy and got to go around to the different islands and play for the service men.

He played with Joe DiMaggio and Hank Greenburg. He played with a lot of the big

league players. He had a good life but he was in the south Pacific and that was not a safe

place to be. I worried about him a lot.

After the spring season I went fishing in Alaska with my Uncle Tony. We fished for six

months from the Excellent. The last of May we fished in Thremek Bay and it was a real

nice season.

I turned 17 years old that July and the experiences I had and the fun of being with all my

relations was great. All of us young guys had fun not being married and all. The old

married crew guys didn't have as much fun that trip and it was hard on them to be away

from their families for 6 months. My uncle fished for 30 years and was home for only one

month each year, December. That year we fished to November, made $800 and came

home to Seattle. We arrived at the fisherman's dock on a Wednesday at 8:30 a.m. and tied the boat up. After all the hugging and kissing was over, the wives were all crying and

such because they were happy, I packed my dirty clothes to head home with. My cousin

Mike, my dad's brother Marco's son, came aboard and had another job on a different

boat for me. The boat was the Jhonnie Boy, a sardine seiner and it was heading for

California. Mike said it was going to San Francisco to do some sardine fishing. They

were leaving in two days so I had time to get home to mom and grandma and have them

wash my clothes. I packed right back up and got back to the new boat to fix up my new

bunk. We left on our new adventure right on time.

We left Seattle on the 12th of November on 1939 and we headed out over the straits of

Juan De Fuca. We got to Neah Bay at Tatoosh Island and we made our way out of the

Port and started down the coast of Washington. There were eight men aboard and the

captain was Andy Vitalich. His brother Johnny, Mike and a fellow named Tony were all

on board.

The seiner was western made in the Puget Sound so it was a good salmon seiner and

dragger. The captain, who was killed a few years later on another seiner, was a nice man.

He was killed when a block broke loose onboard. There was also a cook onboard named

Bacoka, the brother of the owner of the Johnnie Boy, my good friend Girgich and myself

rounded out the crew. Girgich died years later too, of cancer.

We started out and we began our boat watch. There are two men on watch a shift for two

hours a piece on the wheel, two hours checking the engine and the rest of the ship. My

partner was my cousin Mike. (In later years Mike and I spent a lot of time on fishing trips

together.)

We have a thing we call Iron Mike on the ship, it's an automatic steering gear where we put the ship on autopilot. It allows us to set the course and the ship steers itself. When it is on autopilot we just watch for ships, logs and things like that. So the next day when the sun comes up we put out a big fish line to try and catch tuna on our way out. They told us to watch the line. When you bring a young kid aboard the guys are gonna play a joke on him and the young kid this time was me and they did play the joke. We were all eating breakfast about 8 a.m. and the captain told me to check the stern and line. As I checked the line and started yelling that we had a fish on it I started to pull the line in. Most of the crew came on deck to watch and cheer me on as I pulled the "fish" in. They got the dip net all ready and here comes this big gunnysack that they had put on my hook full of water. That sack on the end of the hook was catching a lot of water making it heavier. So all I caught was a sack of water. I was mad as I pulled that sack onboard but afterwards we all had a good laugh.

The day went on and I had to get even with the old guys so I played a gag on them. I played a gag I learned up north. After dinner every night after the table was cleared the guys would start a card game for a few hours. About the time they sat down that night to play I went into the galley to pretend to get a cup of coffee. I dropped a handful of pepper onto the galley stove and shut the door on my way out. A few minutes later they all came pouring out of the galley eyes watering, sneezing, coughing and choking. I was laughing so hard at that sight I was almost falling onto the deck. Of course I said I didn't know anything about it but they knew who did it.

We had a good crew and me, Andy and Girgich became good friends. We were close in age, I was 17, Andy was 21 and Girgich was 22.

We finally got on the coast and it was beautiful trip in calm seas. We were going under

the Golden Gate Bridge and there was San Francisco, the old roaring twenties town.

What a nice site! We tied up on the docks at the foot of the Barbary Coast and it was nice

and sunny. There were pelicans on our deck and everything. It was a whole new

adventure for me.

We fished at night. We left the docks at 3 p.m. in the afternoon and headed out under the

Golden Gate Bridge and out to the ocean. We would wait until dark and then start

running around looking for sardines schools.

The way you fish for sardine is to have a man in the crows nest looking for what looks

like a whole lit up city underwater. The sardine stir around and it looks like light. We call

it fire in the water. We have a big mallet on the bow of the boat and we pound on that on

the deck. If there is a big light flash under the water that means there are fish there so we

let our big seine circle the light in the waters and purse the net up and there they are. We

got up to 100 tons on some nights, but most of the time we pulled in 50-70 tons. Those

were all good nights. We had to head in two or three times to run up the Sacramento

River and drop off the catch. There we would have big suction pipes that would come on

in our hatch and pull the fish out. We would go to bed for just a few hours and then go

back out.

One day we started out and the sea got rough under the bridge and it was too rough to go

out so we turned back and I liked that because we got to go into town. We got to do some

bowling and going through the town. That was like back in the roaring 20's and it was

just as wild as it had been back then. San Francisco was a real exciting town. The full

moon would come up for 7 days each month so the old married men would get in a bus and head home for 8-10 days and leave us young guys to watch the boat. We had a lot of fun but that's another story.

The season went on and we left San Francisco and headed south to fish in San Pedro. It was the last of February and I had spent Christmas and New Years aboard the boat in Frisco. We went further south and fished around Santa Cruz Islands and the Santa Barbara Islands. There was a lot of beautiful ocean in that area. It was also a nice town. I got into bowling and we bowled up to 10 hours a day sometimes. It cost .20 cents a game at that time and me and three buddies had a lot of fun there. It was another great life adventure and memories.

Fishing was finally over in Pedro and I had a chance to go fish tuna in Mexico out to the Galapagos Islands. I went aboard the Elizabeth boat run by A. Zankich. We left Pedro and the first school of tuna we ran into and wanted to fish we were supposed to stand out on the grading side of the boat and hooked the tuna swinging them in. They were 50-70 pound fish and I couldn't do it so I was put in the hatch to freeze tuna as they came down. We piled them like a cord of wood in the hatch. After weeks of being up in the crows nest getting burned by the sun I now had to load tuna and pack it in ice.

A bad storm came up and we started bucking the storm home to Pedro. Pedro was nine days away and our ice machine had broken. We toughed the storm out for 10 days. ~~Forty days later~~ we all got to the cannery and opened our hatch to find our tuna rotten. We ended up selling the whole load for fertilizer and I got paid $40 for 40 days. I bought a bus ticket with that $40 and headed home.

Chapter 4

Now my life was starting to change. The winter finally was over and I got a job in Alaska

fishing for herring with my Uncle Tony. This was my second chance to fish on the big

boat and this time start from the beginning. I was to be the engineer on the 70 foot seine

boat The Paul. The boat was named after a well known old-time fisherman and his

family, a man named Paul Luketa who had passed away. Mrs. Luketa, his widow, had

leased the boat to my uncle for the 1940 herring season in Prince William Sound in

Alaska. I ran the engine, a 135 HP Atlas engine. All I had to do was watch the oil and

check it once a day and I worked the water pumps for wash day. Back then the old time

Atlas diesel engines ran for years without one bit of a problem. They just went on and ran

day and night.

We got the net ready on the deck at Fisherman's wharf and got ready to leave. We would

buy groceries for six months and take a few barrels of wine, home made, with us. We

also carried about 50 chickens. We put them in our skiff and make a cover of old seine

web over them. We had the net in the big hatch and our groceries incases. We also

carried a lot of freight for the cannery, usually machinery, all lashed onto our deck. Our

skiff was up on the stern all tied down and ready to go.

My cousins were all going north, there was the captain Sam Mezich and his boys Arnie,

who died of cancer in 1989, and Walt, who was my age. We had gone to school together

and we pals most of our lives. Walt died of cancer a year after his brother. Their brother

Pete was also onboard; he died when he fell off scaffolding in 1950 and drown. Tony

Scrivnich, my mothers sister's oldest boy, who fished with us for several years and Hank

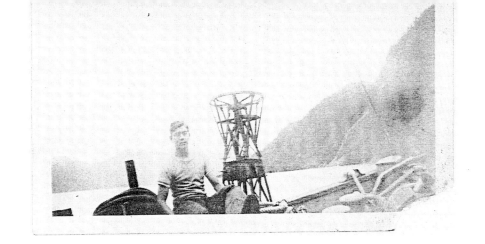

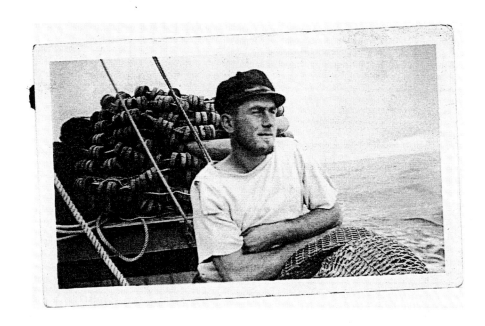

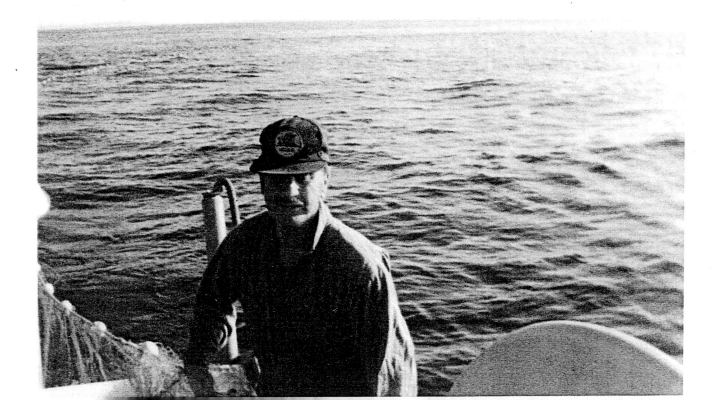

Zuvich who fished with his step dad Martin on the boat. They had a boat named the

Newport and he also owned the boat Daisy. The Mezich family had the Mary M for years

then later they got the biggest boat in the fleet, The Western Chief, an 85 foot seine. This

was all later though so let's get back to my story....

We all left at a certain time, on a certain day every year because the Semon Arrows was a

bad stretch of water. It took us about 30 hours from departing from Seattle so we would

leave to hit that section while it was flooding and then we would zip through those

swirling tide rips in a few hours.

Now we were all ready to leave, all loaded up and ready to go on may 29th at 6 a.m. in the

morning but our last night in town, and we were kind of wild in those days no different

than the young fellow today sowing their oats as they say, before sailing we all went out

to raise a little Cain. We went to a tavern in Garfield Street where the Magnolia Bridge

starts on 15th Ave. There was an owner that didn't like us very well and we had had

problems in the past so we were gonna give him a hard time and then take off. We started

having some fun and it got a bit rough and I remember going into the bathroom and

pulling the whole toilet up off the floor. Water was shooting all over and a few of the

mirror were busted. We all took off, there were about 10 of us and we were all cousins,

and headed for the dock. We got to our boats and got into our bunks to start sleeping it

off. It had been about 2 a.m. when we had come in and when we woke up at 6 a.m. the

dock was full off police. They had heard from someone, or maybe one of us talking about

it, that we were leaving in the morning for fishing up north. They corralled the dock with

about three police cars and then here came our parents, my uncle and captain, the old

timers and their families ready to leave. After some searching the bar owner picked us out and we ended up all on the dock. Because the captain had to leave they police took the

owner aside and talked with him telling him we would not bother him again and that we

would all chip in and pay for the damage. He finally agreed not to press charges and

collected $300 from the skippers. They had bailed us all out but after the others left we

got a good cussing out and a warning from our superiors. We were now an hour late for

our departure too.

We left for Alaska. There were five seiners and after the loved ones said good-bye we left

for the north.

The trip north was a regular routine trip. It took us 7 days and nights and we traveled

steady standing our watches at the wheel. We ate, slept and watched the beautiful sights

along side the passage up the Johnson straits through Canada and up to Ketickan on to

Wrangle Narrows and passage. Petersberg was a real nice little town and there were

many like it quiet and secluded among the mountains. There were waterfalls and all, just

plain pretty country. We usually saw deer along the beaches and we would pick up some

fresh meat for the summer.

As we traveled north we would stop by the Columbia Glacier and go along side some of

the big chunks of ice. We would chop ice in blocks and put it in our ice box, and then

we'd have ice for keeping our fresh meat cold and fresh.

We got to our cannery and unloaded. Finally we would get to start fishing for the herring.

We usually tied up together in bad weather with the other uncles and cousins in some

bay. Usually we chose Mount McLoud Harbor that was the bay on Montague. It had a

beautiful inlets and bays all around it and we would harbor many good memories of the

place, especially me. Crab fishing, octopus catching, duck hunting, deer hunting and bear hunting, it was all here. There were huge brown bears, huge monsters that were all you

needed to live on the bay. A little salt and flour and you could live there forever. I always

wanted to go back because those were the best fishing years of my life and there were

several experiences here that I would never forget. In fact one time the weather was bad

and about four of our boats were tied together at the head of the bay. The old monsoon

made us stay aboard and play pinochle or poker. Those of us young guys couldn't take

the boredom so we decided to go on a big bear hunt. We headed for the beach with our

skiff and we had 22 rifles and a couple of shotguns. We were ready. We headed up the

side of a pretty big hill and the woods were thick. We were gonna get a big bear, up to a

ton we had decided. These brown bears are dangerous but we were all hunters and ready

to get that bear. Off we went further up, then, all a once, there was a crashing sound in

the woods ahead of us. A growl like thunder came from the trees. We were standing there

one minute and then in the next minute we were all running down the hill as fast as we

could, all 7 of us. We headed for the beach tripping over each other until we were all in

the skiff. All of us were scared so badly that we were shaking and out of breath from

running. All the big brave hunters headed back for our boats only to have the old timers

laugh and kid us. The cook, he was waiting with a knife in hand to start carving up our

bear laughing. I will never forget that one.

That time was dangerous but not as dangerous as the time my brother Gus and I went

duck hunting. We went duck hunting on that very same beach with our big heavy seine

skiff. After we had hunted we came back to find our skiff high and dry on the long sandy

beach but the tide was coming in so we weren't worried. We'd just have to wait.

Suddenly this big brown bear started toward us. I was scared and we didn't know what to do. We backed up and backed up but the big brown bear just kept coming at us. He was

coming close because he was more curious than anything else. He was nosy and wanted

to see what the skiff was. We backed out into the water with our hearts pounding. We

were scared to death. We tried to stay as quiet as we could and the big brown bear sniffed

and grunted and then suddenly turned and headed back for the hills. We started breathing

again. I will never forget that day and how scared Gus and I were. It had been a real

experience.

My teen years were coming close to an end now but I felt like I was a man already. I had

traveled all over the ocean from far north to Alaska to way south in the Pacific on toward

Mexico. I traveled the whole ocean yet I had still not been on a train or a plane or inland

in Washington State. I had learned a whole lot of different kinds of fishing, herring, seine

and salmon. And I'd fished a whole lot of different places the Columbia River, Alaska,

Puget Sound, Purse Seine and Gillnette. Now here I was 19 years old and on my way to

fish in Alaska during the season in 1941. On the way home that season everything went

okay. We had had a nice season and the good old ship Paul was in good shape. The crew

was glad to arrive on Fisherman's Wharf and all our loved ones were on the dock to meet

us. After all the hugging, kissing and crying was over we headed home to my mom and

brothers and another winter in Seattle.

Chapter 5
1941 – A Whole New Life Experience

Upon coming home from the north, about one week later, I got a job as a deck hand and cook aboard the boat The Newport with my cousin Oren Basihoi and Captain Martin Suich. Dragging, another form of fishing is a whole new adventure in fishing. The fishing is bottom fishing and it is on the ocean out past Neah Bay Tattosh Isle which is the last piece of land you see when going out to sea. Beyond that is the rest of the world. Draggers carry a net that has two wings on the front end and a long tube on the back like a net and a sack on the back part of the wings with a based ring bottom that fish can be let out of. There are two doors we call a let-down on the bottom of the boats tow. This net sets and then drags on the bottom for several miles then we drum up the net and the doors come up first, then the wings and then we boom up the net and up comes up to five tons of fish. We catch tons of red snapper, sole and up to 50 other different kinds of fish. We also get octopus fish, wolf fish, dog fish and even salmon and halibut, it is real interesting fishing. We load up sometimes on the dog fish which we take and cut the livers out of. The livers are used to make vitamin E pills. We get a good price for the livers too. We caught up to 7 drums. The drums are 250 lbs and we used to get up to $1 a pound and that was good money in 1941. We would load up to 60,000 pounds per week and we would leave home early Sunday at about 3 p.m. and run 12 hours on the straits to the ocean and drag all week. We would stop at dark in the evening and then we would start again the next morning. I was the cook and I used to buy 25 big steaks, lettuce, 20 heads and potatoes. We would have steak, potatoes and salad. I'd make fish meals in between.

One day I was on the Newport with my cousin Martin and there was a 100 mile an hour
wind blowing. We were dragging under the Tacoma Narrows Bridge. We had to clean
dog fish for their livers and the price was $3.50 a pound, which was especially good in
those days. I was making good money $300 dollars a week or more. It was then that one
of the scariest experiences of my life took place. We had dropped anchor and the wind
was blowing pretty hard. We were about a ½ mile from the bridge and we heard a terrible
rumble like thunder. We looked over and there was the bridge going down. What a sight
that high monster of a bridge was collapsing in front of our eyes. I had a small camera
and I took a few pictures but the captain said, boys we'd better pick up anchor ad head
home. This was very scary and the seas were mean and rough. We went on our way to
Seattle but what a storm that was. I think about it today and I still can't believe that I was
there the day the bridge fell.

We had caught a lot of dog fish in the west pass area so we kept going back. We got more
than a few good loads out of there. It was December and almost Xmas and it was cold.
We took another trip down to the Narrows Bridge to fish for dog fish and it was
December 7, 1941 at about 9:30 a.m. when the news cut in there was nice church music
playing on the radio. The news was that we were being attacked by the Japanese at Pearl
Harbor. The Harbor was being bombed and that meant that we were going to war and we
all knew it. I was just 20 years old and I knew that meant I was probably going to have to
go. I was scared but so was everybody else in the world. Germany was taking over
Europe, Japan was trying to take us over and the whole world was in a terrible mess.
My mother had three sons and she was a widow but Gus got drafted and went into the
Navy. He ended up in the South Pacific where the war was really tough. A lot of guys

died on the Mariana's and at Guadla Canal. My brother Mike was a ball player with the

New York Giants and he went into the Navy as a specialist in the athletic department and

played baseball on most of the islands in the South Pacific. He was on the team

DiMaggio and Ted Williams, as well as most of the other top baseball players, were on.

They were players from the big leagues and they played for the service men. He was

lucky to make it home as did my brother Gus. As for me I got the greatest experience of

my life, four years in the United States Navy aboard an old four stacker Destroyer DD

231-Uss Hatfield. At first both my brothers were in the war so I tried to get a 6 month

deferment because my mother would have been alone. Besides I was in the fishing

business and there was a need for fishermen.

My mother and I went to the draft board which consisted of a 5 man board in the armory

in the center of Seattle where the World's Fair was later held in 1961. We walked into the

board meeting and there was this big man Mr. Blackstock there. He was the head of the

draft board. My mother and I explained our situation, she being a widow who could not

read and write with no way to take care of herself. She needed one of her boys home to

take care and help her. With me being a fisherman and the need for fishermen to catch

fish to feed the troops we pleaded with the board but Mr. Blackstock said there was not a

chance of me getting out of the draft. I had to take my physical that day and the next

morning I would be sworn into the army. My mom cried and pleaded with the fat pig but

he said no way, tomorrow you come in. We left and I thought that after being a seaman

all my life there was no way I was going into no army. So I made arrangement s and two

days later I sworn into the Navy. The day after I was sworn in the mail man brought us

our mail and said there was an important thing from the army and here was the deferment for 6 months. I took it and ran over to the 13ᵗʰ Navel District on pier 91. I went in and

saw the head Naval officer and showed him the deferment. I said I can't go into the

Navy, I got a deferment and he said son you are in the Navy and no way are you getting

out now. You joined, he said, and you were sworn in, you're a navy man now.

I was so mad and furious; I went straight to the armory and charged in. Blackstock and

the board members were all there and I went right up to Blackstock and told his fat face

off. I told him that my mom had cried to get him to give me a leave but he had said no

way, you're in the army. I tore up the deferment card and threw it in his face. I told him

that if I got killed in the service I would come back and haunt him the rest of his life. I

stormed out leaving them there with their mouths open.

The next day I was to leave for Bremerton for Navy training. I felt bad because we had

left poor mom at home in her little house alone with no kids. All three of her boys were

off to war and could be killed. I can't imagine what must have been going through her

heart and mind. What suffering that must have been? With all of us in the service she

could have been left completely alone with no one to help her read and write anything.

My heart breaks still every time I think of what she had to suffer. She's at rest now so I

know she is in heaven. But then here I was in Bremerton waiting to see what would

happen next. Where was I going? I'll tell you I was a nervous wreck. I just wondered day

after day but on the sixth day of August I got the news and orders to pack my gear. We

were headed for the war.

Chapter 6
The Beginning of World War II

We headed for Paine Field. We were put on a bus in Bremerton and all the windows were painted black but it got us to the field. We were given a box of rations and put on an army plane. We were all just boys, on the plane we spread out. The plane took off. The windows on the plane were painted black to so none of us knew where we were going. Some of the guys started trying to scratch the paint off the windows to try and see where we were going. I took a look out through the space they had scratched and saw nothing but blue ocean so I told the boys that we were headed south but God know where. Five hours later we landed and the doors opened. We were at an air force base in Honolulu, Hawaii. We saw Pearl Harbor, man what an awful sight. Another bus with black windows picked us up and dumped us off at a half destroyed dock. The next thing we knew we were aboard the battle wagon the USS Nevada. We were told to get in line and they put us in crews. We then had lunch which was pork chops, vegetables and a can of pop. After that they told us to go to bed because we had a big day ahead of us the next day. I heard an engine running all night. The next day we were woke up at 6 a.m. and found we were underway.

We had a breakfast of powdered eggs and slices of tough bacon. Afterwards we were all tied with a line and given hard hats with lights on the front of them. In the Double Bottom of the ship there are 2304 compartments. We were all told to stick together because if any of us got lost we might never be found. We were given plastic bags and there were big holes in the decks above us. If a bomb was dropped down where we were it would blow the ship apart. A lot of guys were killed down there in the first attack. We now had to go through the bottom decks and pick up pieces of flesh. Some guys found

fingers and parts of legs. We had little masks on to help us breathe but it still stunk. We

had to do this for five days. About 70 of us ended up with diphtheria and landed in sick

bay. When we got to Bremerton I spent five days in the hospital. Most of the guys didn't

get sick and ended up heading for the South Pacific right away. When my call came I was

sent to Pier 91 in Seattle and got aboard a Destroyer, the USS Hatfield. Little did I know

this would be my home for the next four years. I was a seaman 1st class

There are many Television shows about the war but very few, or hardly any, television

shows, books or movies were shown about the war of the north, the Aleutian Islands off

Adak, Kiska A Michitka Islands, Attu, Dutch Harbor and the Kodiak Islands. My story is

true and what a great war was fought in the Aleutians. They were occupied by Japanese

troops.

This part of my story is dedicated to the men lost aboard our ship and the medals we got

and earned for the action the Grand Old Lady and her crew went through in the four years

of World War II that I served.

The Grand Old Lady

She was an old four stacker. The USS Hatfield was a destroyer in the United States Navy.

She had four stacks and four big guns, one forward, one amid ship, one starboard upper

deck and one portside upper deck. The last of these is called the well deck. She had 6

twenty millimeter guns, two port and starboard side of the bridge and two amid ship just

aft of the big gun. There were also two guns in the bathtub. It was a big bathtub

approximately 30 feet long and 15 feet wide. It stood 10 feet up from the deck and it was

four feet deep with two millimeter guns back to back. There were four torpedoes, two

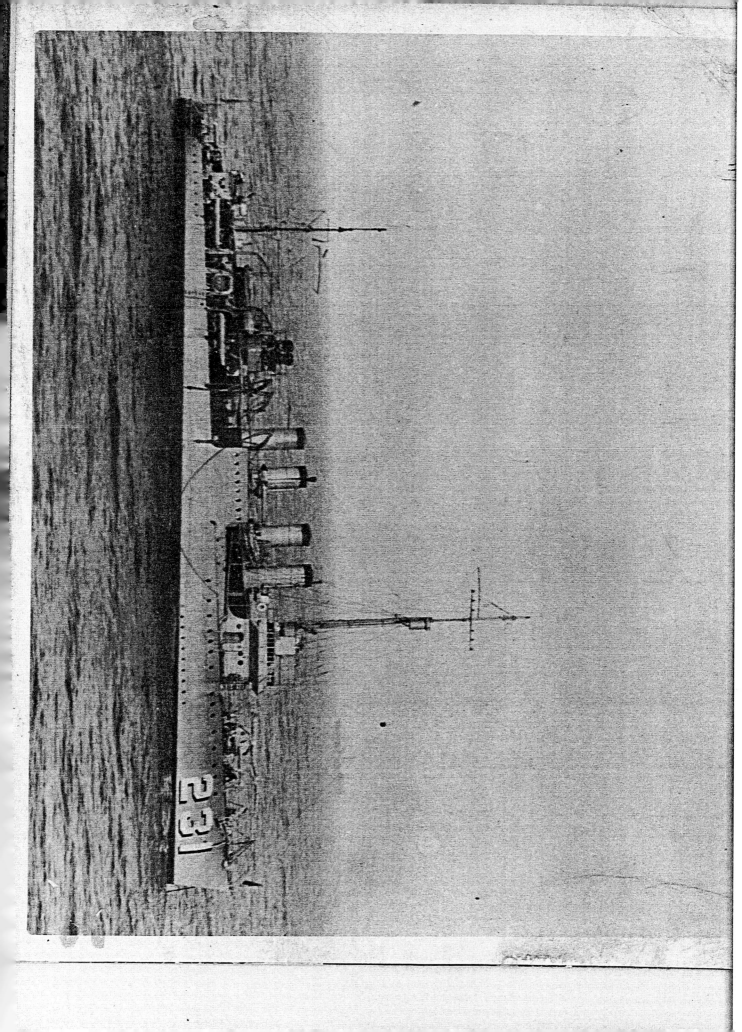

starboard and two port. These were on the main deck and she had four depth charge guns

on the starboard side and four on the port side of the ship. We also had 24 depth charge

cans that rolled off her stern. All in all she had three big guns, six twenty millimeter, four

torpedoes and thirty depth charge cans and all of it could be let go at the same time.

Her forward compartment was the chain locker for the big old fashion anchor on deck,

and then came the paint locker. The next compartment was the slight bunk petty officer

compartment, then came the seaman's quarters with eighty bunks and then ten more for

Chief Boson stewards or as we called them "sea going bellhops". There was only one

companion way to the deck hatch for the entire forward seaman to get out of general

quarters. It was a mess getting up and out only one person at a time. Then we had the

ammunition compartment and that was next to the seaman's quarters. Going aft of the

ship next was the fire rooms and the pressured compartment room; they were next to each

other. The fire room was huge.

The water tanks came next. We made our own water from sea water. Then there were our

big fuel tanks all in compartments below deck. The fire meant seamen, or as we called

them, the snipers, came next. I don't know why we called them snipers. There were

eighty-five of them.

Above deck the first compartment was the doctors' state room. Above top deck were the

officers' quarters and the captains' stateroom. The quartermasters chart room, sound

room, radar room and forward room came next and the bridge was on the top deck.

That's where the steering lookouts out on the flying bridge are. Then aft of the bridge is a

space of thirty feet only a stack goes up from the middle of the well deck starboard side

and portside were the companion way in the middle of these was the gunnery stack that had all the rifles. This had all our rifles, machine guns, forty-five pistols and grenades as well as other arsenal.

Next was the main part of the stomach, the galley where all our food is cooked and served. You can get to there from all parts of the ship by the stewards. Toward the stern was our big freezer which held months of food, meat etc. and next to that was our potato locker as we called it, all the cases of fruit and vegetables of all kinds were there. These were supposed to last for several months as well. Our torpedoes took up space from our galley back to the john. The john, or bathroom, had showers, six stools, six urinals. We had one half day for firemen and the other half for seaman. We were only allowed five minutes on account of the water shortage. Behind the restrooms on our fantail were the twenty-four depth charges.

I was enthralled with the ship for many reasons. My grandfather had been an officer aboard a huge battle ship. We were of Austrian decent and my grandfather served under the Kaiser at the time he was on the ship. He was in the navy too when he came to the United States in the late 1800's. He became a commercial fisherman. The love of the seas was in my blood.

Having been a fisherman up north before the war the navy made me a seaman 1st class. Because I had fished from Nome, Alaska to Mexico I was considered an old hat at living at sea. I was sworn in as a seaman 1st class into the 13th Navel District, I guess they thought I wouldn't need any training, boy were they wrong.

When I saw my name on the bulletin board for the Hatfield I had pictured in my mind a big new destroyer. When I got off the bus and saw the old 4 stacker from the last war I was surprised.

Whe I got on board I was met by a 260 lb. man named Van Sweringer from Kansas City,

Missouri. First thing he asked me was do you smoke. I said no way and he explained that

the ship was full of ammunition from bow to stern. That ship was a bomb leaving for

Dutch Harbor in Alaska. We left as soon as the captain came aboard. Sweringer

explained that there were no bunks in up forward in the seamen's quarters so at that time

they would put me aft in the fireman's quarters. He took me back aft on this hatchway

that was so tight that I could hardly fit sea bag and all. In the stops he got me a bunk

above cases of ammunition with four big steam pipes above me that cracked and made

noises all night. It was so bad and I was so scared that I had my rosary out. I could hardly

hear myself praying.

When the skipper came aboard we left at once, 30 knots full flank speed. All I heard was

that they hoped subs didn't hit us with the load we had or that those Japanese planes

didn't come at us. I was very scared that first night and I don't think I slept in the first

couple of hours either. I kept waiting for something to happen.

The morning came at 6 a.m. and I was up and out on the deck. We were just leaving the

straits and were cruising off Vancouver Island. I was taken to the seamen's quarters and

had breakfast on top of cases of ammunition used as a table. I met a few of the crew then,

Chief Boson mate Angelo, a nice Italian man and Chief Boson Cossy, I could never say

his name but we became very close friends. He was pretty cool and tall, 6 feet. He

weighed 185 lbs and he was all muscle but no brains. But he was pretty tough and I was

19 years old and a rock. Cossy was always testing me. We would bet on wrestling around

and he would try and take me on at other times. He never won. We had a real nice

friendship. Most of the guys were 20 years old and in for five years or more but there was this one guy, our head officer Chief Garrett who was a tough old salt. He must have

already been in the navy for 20 years or more. He was all navy and when he yelled out

orders we all jumped. The captain was a man called Vaness. He was very nice and knew

his business. Our executive officer was Mr. Dodds, he kept to his quarters. The officers

and the captain were seen mostly when they were on duty on the bridge. There was a

little officer, what we called a 90 day wonder, who came out of college with an officer

ensign rating. His name was Mr. Cullen, but more about him later.

Chief Bosn barked at me in his gruff voice, Budnick get up to the executive office, Mr.

Dodds wants to see you right now. Boy I was more than a little nervous. I got up to the

Exec. Office and knocked. A gruff voice said come in and I stepped in, saluted and stood

at attention. He finally said, "relax we're not much for navy rules here with this damn

war going on. We have to be on alert at all times". He went on asking me what I did

before the war. I told him about my fishing experiences in Alaska, California and Mexico

and he asked what my job had been on the tuna boat in Mexico. I told him that they

always put the young guys with good eyes up in the crows nest looking out for tuna.

When I yelled that I'd seen tuna the crew would jump out of their bunks or stop what

they were doing, put on their boots and grab their poles to get ready for the tuna. He said,

you know a lot about the bays and all up in Alaska huh? I said yes and he told me that I

could help. He said my first job was up in the crows nest. This was about 10 a.m. and he

told me they needed my eyes. He told me that at 1 p.m. I was to climb into the crows nest

and use spy glasses to report everything I saw. He said to report every log I saw too

because I didn't know what a periscope looked like. He did tell me that when I saw my

first one though I would never forget it for the rest of my life. He told me to go have my lunch and then get up in the nest. He also said he wanted to hear more of my fishing

stories too. He told me I looked like a good hard working young man and said we would

get a long just fine and then he dismissed me. So I went to Chief Garrett and told him

what I was told to do. He came up with a few of his talks, he said that the crows nest is

seventy feet up and that when the ship started bucking in heavy seas we list over so far

we dip water in the crows nest. Sometimes the guys that man the crows nest forget to tie

themselves on and that, he said, was a bad thing.

He went on with some more stories of funny things that happened. Here is what happened

to the last sailor we lost.

The ship was icing on badly and we were in 40 below freezing. The ship was listing with

ice and bucking the sea real bad. When you man the crows nest you know to wear your

headphones at all times. The chief listened in his headphones but could not hear a thing

from the guy in the nest so he had figured that his headphones had froze, which they

often do. He sent another man up with his headphone and when the guy got there he

called back to say the other guy must have flipped out on a big swell because he didn't

see him but his phones were there. The chief told the man to send down the headphones

and he did and gave them to me. Low and behold the man's voice came through the

phones and he was saying, I'm jumping out to sea because it has got to be warmer than it

is up here.

The chief told me good luck, gave me my phones and a special spy glass and said, keep

your eyes open up there. He said I had a couple 100 men depending on me and wished

me luck. I headed up, a little nervous and a little scared. It is a long way up there. It was

farther up than on a tuna clipper. I got up there in the nest and put my phones on to test them with the bridge and they worked. I hung my spy glass over my neck and started my

first watch ever aboard the big ship. Boy the Old Lady looked good from up there. I felt

like the king of the mountain. The ship skimmed the sea like a knife. Lucky for my first

duty the weather was calm. The first call I made was a porpoise off the bow. They were

racing us, having a little fun. The first hour went real nice. We were about 20 miles off

the northern tip of Vancouver and it was a little foggy or cloudy maybe. What happened

next happened so quickly it caught me off guard. A plane came out of the clouds. I

started yelling into the phone that there was a plane starboard side up ahead. They were

yelling back at what angle, what position. I was yelling back up in the sky starboard side,

can't you guys see it, it's so plain, its one of our OBY. I was yelling down to the bridge

and pointing up to the plane and the last thing I heard from the bridge was, 'get down

here right now and report to the executive officer at once boy". I was scared because I

wasn't sure what I did. I thought I had done well but when I entered Mr. Dodd's

stateroom he was very unhappy. He said you know Mr. Budnick you endangered the

whole ship. He said you have the crow's nest that has position angle right there. Didn't

you take training in camp, he asked. I said no sir and I explained that my having been at

sea all my life they didn't seem to feel I needed training. I explained that my eyes were

good and that I did spot the plane as it broke through the clouds. He said that those were

very good skills but it was not navy standard so he said I'd have to go to school down in

the Boson Chief's quarters. He gave me a blue jacket manual to study until we got back

to Seattle and then he said he would give me a test. He asked me how I was with the

wheel and I told him I could stay at the wheel for hours. He said well, you may have to.

He asked if I got sea sick and I said no sir. He told me to report to Ensign Cullen and he would schedule me. I said yes sir. He told me to study hard and said he hoped to not see

me in his office until we got back to sea. He said dismissed and I said thank you sir,

saluted and left. Boy I was glad to get out and breathe some fresh air. The blue manual he

gave me is the navy's bible. Just take a quick look through it I told myself but when I

looked I thought no way, I am going to have to study. All those signals and flags, there

were a million things to learn. I hate studying.

I reported to the bridge with Mr. Cullen who showed me all that I was to do while on the

wheel. The steering wheel was a big round wheel, five feet across, made of two actual

wheels that were brass. They have two compasses that were completely different than I

was use to. You stand on a platform one foot high. The wheel came up to my upper chest.

A big arrow ahead of the wheel points to numbers. When they bark orders like five points

starboard you get to that arrow. Things worked out and I was on the wheel for two hours

then I switched with a quarter master and stood out on the fly bridge with binoculars for

two hours looking for periscopes, planes or whatever. So my first shift on the bridge was

over with Mr. Cullen saying, very good shift Mr. Budnick.

I slept with eighty other seaman on the forward facile but what the navy didn't know was

that I talked in my sleep. I yelled something on the fifth night, I guess with all the

excitement I got excited, I gave out a scream and started yelling something and boy all

eighty seamen jumped out of their bunks. Some were running up the hatchway because

they thought we were being attacked. Everybody on the ship head about my problems so

Chief Garrett finds me and says why don't you just move in with me? He also said Mr.

Dodds, the executive officer, wanted to see me. I told him thanks chief and once again

I'm standing in front of executive officer Dodds. He is second in command aboard the ship. He says Mr. Budnick I didn't expect to see you again until we got to Seattle. When

you joined the navy did you tell them you had nightmares and screamed and yelled in

your sleep? You got the whole forward crew on this ship shaking and ready for action. If

we were in Seattle right now, he said, you would get a discharge you know that. He got

the phone in his hand and called on the loud speaker for Mr. Garrett, chief boson, to

report to Dodd's stateroom on the double. Mr. Garrett walked in and saluted. Mr. Dodds

says what do we do with this fisherman here. Mr. Garrett grinned and said, well we could

throw him over the side and our problems would be over. Mr. Dodds said, well that's an

idea then we can fight the rest of this war in peace. Any other ideas Chief, he asked.

"Yes", Mr. Garrett said, "I think I can solve this problem sir, besides we may need his

experience in the waters off Alaska. As I understand it we will be fighting in the

Aleutians for the next few years or so".

Mr. Dodds says well, we'll see what happens in the future, take this fisherman and shape

him up, he said, he's all yours. Mr. Garrett and I salute and left. Once on deck again the

chief tells me to follow him. We headed for the gunnery shack. I thought that maybe he

was going to shot me or something like that. We got to the gunnery shack which was on

the main deck. The compartment was twenty feet in length and ten foot wide. The chief

said nothing, he was studying something. I had no idea what he was thinking. He finally

turns to me and says go down to the fire room to the machine shop and tell the machinist

1st class James that I want to see him now if he isn't busy. He wasn't so we went back to

the gunnery shack. When we got there the chief says to James, can we move this rack of

guns over to this wall and put a bunk on this wall and locker up here? James pulls out his

measuring tape and does some measuring and then says it can be done chief. Garrett asks

James could it be done today so we can all get some sleep tonight. James says it will be done in three to four hours. The chief says thank you Mr. James when we get back from sea I'll buy you a drink. It's a deal, James said. So I had lunch and went back to the wheel. I finished my shift at 1600 hours and Mr. Cullen says, you better move, so I went down to my old bunk and packed my sea bag up. I moved to my new quarters and that's were I lived for the next four years. It was the best bunk on the ship; they called it the Budnick Shack. A couple of the boson mates and a couple of seamen installed a heater in there and put in a table and a hot plate. My shack ended up being a coffee shop. I made bacon and eggs in there and for the four years it ended up being a hang out for anyone who wanted to be there.

My shack was next door to the galley so a lot of stuff disappeared from the galley but the cooks knew where it was going, in fact a few times a week the cooks would stop in for a good meal.

We finally came into Dutch Harbor and we were on full alert. We were all very nervous men aboard that ship. All we needed now was for the Japanese to come and drop bombs on us as we were unloading. There must have been a couple of thousand cases of ammunition and a lot of big stuff that we had on deck that had to be unloaded. We were actually several miles out of Dutch Harbor. Suddenly the speaker boomed out, Budnick report to the bridge on the double. I said to myself, now what did I do? I got there and the captain was on the bridge. I was a little shaken but I saluted. The captain asked if I had ever been or fished out of here. I said yes that I had been there several times. He told me to stand by. He said if there were any moves that they made wrong while they were docking I should just yell out. I said yes sir. It all went fine although it wasn't that big a dock. The skipper got her in there just fine. I did tell the captain what happened to us

when we were tied up to the dock. A wind hits in there called a willow. It blasts through

like a whirlwind. I told him we were tied up all night. One season we were hit in the

middle of the night. It broke all our lines off the dock. We barely got the engine going

before we ended up on the beach. The captain said we wanted to get out of there as soon

as we unloaded. He said we also didn't want to get trapped by Japanese in here so we got

unloaded and then got orders to report to Bangor, Washington to load up for our own use.

We had a straight run and our course was from Dutch Harbor to Tatoosh Island down the

straits of San Juan De Fuca into our ammunition depo at Bangor. The trip back was a

little rough with winds at 55 knots and seas with 15-20 foot swells. I thought nothing

about that as our ship was so big we cut through the swells and we were like a sub most

of the time. I did spend a lot of time on the steering wheel, as most of the ships crew was

sea sick and I took three shifts straight on the wheel.

Chapter 7
The First Action

Our home base was Pier 91, the 13th Naval District, which was no more than two miles

from my home where my mother lived in her small home. My mom paid five dollars a

month for rent and I had $20 a month taken out of my pay while the navy added another

$22 so my mom had $42 a month to live off of. We landed at Pier 91 and tied up the ship.

I was happy and I wanted to run home and see my mom. I couldn't go though because we

had a starboard and port watch. I was the new man on board so I had to stand watch for

four hours and then load groceries for another four hours. I went to see Dodds and he said

I couldn't go. I begged but he said there had to be a full crew of men to handle the ship in

case of an emergency. He let me make a phone call though and I called home. My mom

cried. I was the first of her three sons she had heard from in several months. She was very

glad I was still alive. I was not allowed to say where we were going, (I didn't know either

though), so it was a short phone call. She asked if I had heard from my two brothers, they

were both in the South Pacific in action, I told her no. I told her that she would get letters

from them soon. I had to hang up and I thanked Mr. Dodds and went up on deck. I

dropped a few tears thinking of my poor mom.

We got orders to take off the next morning and head for the strait of San Juan DeFuca.

We would have a plane PBY towing a sleeve; it was about 40 feet long and round like a

tube. We had to take turns on our twenty mill guns. My turn came up and they put me in

the harness. When the sleeve came by we started shooting, boy it was pretty exciting. The

plane was towing a big target behind him and he was a good mile away. Not knowing

that much about the guns I was standing out on the deck looking out and I didn't see the

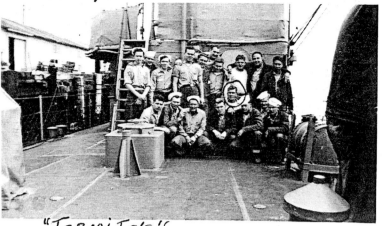

MY - GANG - 1945.

"TERMITE'S"

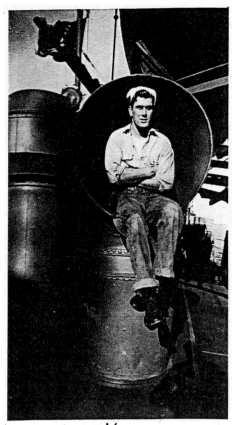

LASY

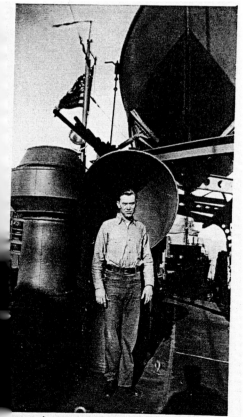

KANSAS - TEX.

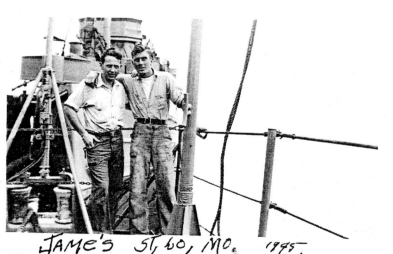

JAME'S ST, LO, MO. 1945.

big gun swing around and out about twenty feet above my head. The last thing I heard

was the captain announcing commence firing. There was a blast over my head and then

this scorching blast of heat that knocked me off my feet and back about twenty feet up

against one of our stacks. I also remember my last scream, it was mama. I thought I had it.

The scream was heard and one of the cooks, Jimmy Boy. (He fell over board a year later

and we lost him) I woke up in the doctors' cabin, or as it was called by some of the

sailors, the Butchers Shop. My face was all black and burned and I had some kind of

grease the doc had put on the skin. I could not hear for several days and I kept in sick bay

for twenty-four hours. I was teased for days. I was a casualty. When we practiced I was

told to put in ear plugs and stay away from the big gun since that was the gunners' mates'

job.

So far I've been in the way and pulling some dumb stunts. I was doing okay on my

seaman's' shift though. While we were in port for the two days earlier I had to take my

exam. Dodds put me in the chief's quarters and there's the seaman's quarters right next to

it. Dodds gave me an hour to answer 120 questions and then left. My friends helped me a

lot though. I flipped notes out to them and they sent notes back in to me and I passed my

first test with the biggest score I ever got even in all my years in school. I'll never forget

when Dodds called me to his cabin and told me I got a 91 on my test. I was glad it was

over.

Chapter 8
At War

Nobody aboard the ship except the officers knew where we were going or what was next.

We call it scuttlebutt, some said we were headed for the South Pacific or to the Aleutian

islands. The Japanese had taken over the islands of Kiska, Amichitka, Adack and Attu.

We were loaded with ammunition and food and were ready for several months at sea. We

were ready for battle too.

The first thing that happened was that four ships were heading toward us from Canada.

They were British Corvettes. It was the first time I had ever seen anything like them.

They were half our size but just as fast. They had smaller guns but they were fighting

ships. So here we were just circling around in the ocean, waiting for something to happen.

Soon we were joined by two other ships from Seattle, destroyer just like us. The other

destroyers were the USS King and the USS Cain. With the arrival of the two new

destroyers we figured something really big was going to happen. There were 7 ships now

and I was at the wheel. My shift was coming to dusk and I asked Cullen what was up. He

said, you'll see in due time. After a while we found out that we were going to have a

general quarters drill to see how fast we could get into our positions and to our guns.

When this happens, each station reports in to the bridge and it is timed. The G.O. sounded

and I was relieved of the wheel and at my 20 mil gun in minutes, ear phones on and

reporting that starboard gun was ready. We ended up having three drills that night. Boy

was I tired. At 2400 hours I was relieved of my post so I went to my shack and fell dead

asleep. My shift was not on again until 8 a.m. so I slept like a log/ I woke up feeling the ship really traveling. I got out on deck and what a sight. There were five destroyers, four

corvettes and seven big liberty ships. We were in a big convoy. We were zig zagging in

front of those ships. They do fourteen knots so we have to go twenty-eight knots. We

were going back and forth in front of them and it was just a sight. The corvettes were

running along side of the big liberty ships. We were in front of the three destroyers and

two were astern of the convoy. I got to go to breakfast and then reported to the bridge for

my wheel watch. Captain Van Ness, Dodds, Cullen and the quarter master were all on the

wheel. A big discussion was going on and I was told to stand fast. The meeting went on

for five minutes and I was real worried and wondering what I had done wrong now. The

captain and Dodds, the two top men on the ship, spoke to me and I got cold chills. I was

waiting for a punishment but instead he said, Seaman Budnick we have 7 ships with

thirty-five hundred or more marines, Seabees and soldiers aboard. That's over 25

thousand men, he said. It is up to us to deliver them to some of our bases in Alaska safe

and sound. We need your eyes, he said, we want you to get up in the crows nest and do

your very best. All I could say was yes sir and salute. Mr. Cullen took me to his cabin and

said dress heavy it may get cold up there and hold on as we may turn very sharp on these

zig zag courses. He laughed and said I've heard when ships like ours listed badly.

Sometimes we may dip water in the crows nest. He gave me my ear phones and

binoculars around my neck. I stopped by my shack and got a dozen of my sucker candies

and went up the 70 feet to the nest and boy what a sight. The ships were all going

different directions zig zagging, what a sight. Everybody was on alert. This was part of

the 7th Infantry Division and we were convoying so I was looking with my binoculars real

hard for the periscope of a Japanese sub or anything I spotted on my first watch. I spotted

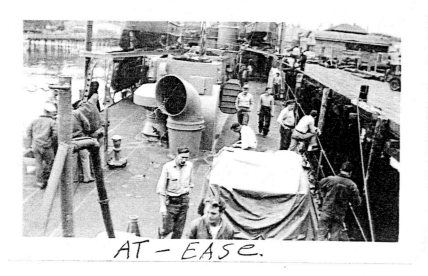

AT - EASE.

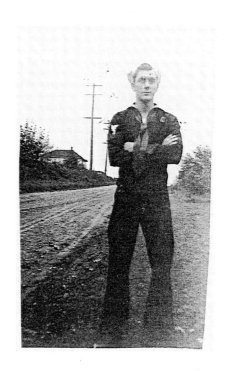

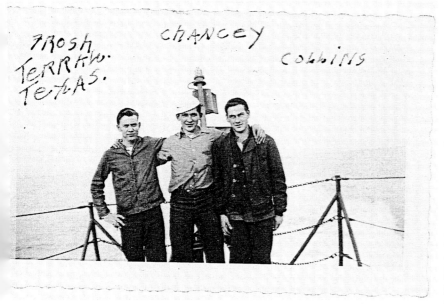

FROSH
TERRAW.
TEXAS.

CHANCEY

COLLINS

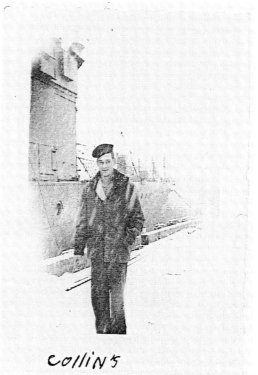

COLLINS

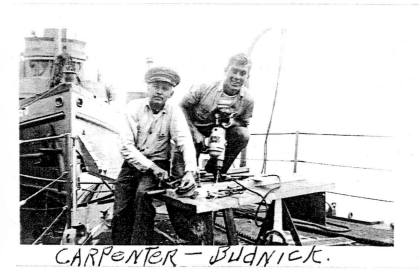

CARPENTER - BUDNICK.

several logs and a porpoise. I got the bridge all ready for general quarters and I saw

something and reported seeing something that no one on the bridge saw. I was scared but

soon, thank God, it was a whale. It blew and its tail came out of the water and showed.

He came up again and again in front of the convoy. Again from the bridge came a

response, very good Mr. Budnick.

Aboard this ship were sailors from Kansas City, Arkansas and all over back in the

Midwest. A lot of the guys had southern accents and they all said I talked funny. There

was Collins, Aines, Schimit and Clark. There were 60 guys, all nice. Woodward was the

preacher; he comes in later in the story.

The trip had my buddies asking me to stand their watch. They were all seasick, lying

around the deck. I felt real sorry for them especially when food was served. I would have

pork chops and these guys were in their bunks that were almost over the long tables we

ate on. They would cuss me. I would eat bacon and eggs in the a.m. and there would be a

steady stream of sailors going up the companion way so I took the wheel, watches and

my crows nest watch almost every day. I would put up to eight hours in on the wheel plus

four hours in the crows nest. All the crew was good friends of mine. The officers aboard

were amazed at the stamina I had. It was all due to the commercial fishing I did where we

were all up looking for fish for ten to twenty hours.

We stopped off in Kodiak. We stood by while a couple of troop ships unloaded. The next

stop was Dutch Harbor and we dropped off the rest of the marines, army soldiers and

Seabees. For the next six months we convoyed ships to the islands that were occupied by

the Americans but the rumors were coming fast and we heard that Admiral Nimitz and

his 2nd Battalion Marines were coming up. Meanwhile Japanese were coming into the

Aleutians with battle wagons, carriers, cruisers and subs. The whole crew was getting real

worked up. While we were on one of our trips with troops north we had several

encounters with subs. When there was contact with a Japanese sub all the ships would go

into general quarters for down smoke screens around our troop ships. Several destroyers

would take after the sub dropping depth charges several times. We chased subs. There

were some great stories on our ship.

Chapter 9
Family Encounters

Last convoy we fueled up and loaded with groceries and ammunition. We were waiting

for our convoy ships to come out of Seattle. It was a nice morning, it was calm and the

sun was out. I was lookout on the bridge, when looking on the straits, we were in between

Port Townsend and Port Angeles, coming along on the ocean was this commercial fishing

boat. When I looked closer I recognized my Uncle Tony who was captain of the boat I

had fished on. My uncle Tony started me on a fishing career when I was in my young

teens. The captain was on the bridge and I took a big chance and approached him. I said

Sir, how would you like to have fresh fish for dinner tonight? I explained that the boat

belonged to my uncle and we could stop him and he would be honored to give us fish.

The captain said we had time to kill and maybe he would stop. We edged closer to the

beach and to the boat the Reliance. We got fairly close and gave a toot on our whistle. At

once I saw his prop stopped and the boat was just drifting. We got close and Mr. Cullen

got on the megaphone. He yelled come along side and my uncle pulled up along our low

midship. I was just twenty feet from him and I yelled hi uncle. Tears welled up in my

eyes as I was like his son. I lived with him and fished with him for years. I fished with

him again years later until he passed away. We got to talking and were glad to see each

other. I told him we could stand some fresh fish so he opened his hatch and got a brailer

hooked up and a couple of his crew started pitching fish in the brailer. Most of our crew

was all on the side asking questions of my uncle about the fish, what kind and he and I

both explained. We explained how beam trolling was done. We took on about 300 lbs of

sole, red snapper and halibut. They dumped it right on our deck which is hot being that the broiler room being below. That was all we took. I yelled to him in front of a couple

hundred men, love you unk. As he pulled away I see a big hanky of his go up to his eyes.

From the bridge on a bull horn came our captains salute and he yelled over to my uncle

good luck. Uncle Tony waved to our captain and gave him a salute as he pulled away.

That was an encounter I'll never forget. (Uncle Tony's son Larry was on a troop ship in

the South Pacific. He did come home after the war)

Our ships showed up and we got under way. We had fresh fish for dinner for two days. I

had to help the cooks clean and get the fish ready. The crew loved it. Every bit of it was

eaten. Uncle Tony had told us there was a big storm coming and there was gonna be

rough seas. He was right. We met our British Corvettes and destroyers just out of Tatoosh

Island and we started our zig zag course. I had first watch in the crows nest and I tell you

our ship was almost under water all the time. Looking down on the ship all you could see

is green water. You couldn't see the deck. Boy it was bad weather with wind 50-55 knots.

The seas were an easy 20 foot swells. It was a miserable trip. There were only a few men

on board who weren't sick the whole trip north. I must have been on the wheel or in the

nest or on the bridge fifteen hours a day but we got good news, I was told by the

executive officer Mr. Dodds and Ensign Cullen that when we got back to port I was to

take the exam for coxswain. I was very happy.

The trip north with our convoy had two general quarters, one we were mostly all asleep

except the men on watch. We got the sounding that there was a sub or something

underwater. It was probably a whale or something. Because it was dark we couldn't be

sure so we dropped six depth charges at 50 feet and didn't see anything. We got back to

the convoy and we had to stay at G.O. for four hours after that. It was a tough night. The winds were up to 40 knots and the seas were 15 feet high. You have to respect the ocean

because it can get plenty mean most of the time. Being on the wheel I kind of glanced at

the gyroscope and figured out our course and I kind of mentioned to Chuck North, the Lt.

on board our ship and a 20 year officer. He said to keep the heading for Dutch Harbor.

Mr. North just grinned and figured I pretty much knew what our next stop would be. Two

days later the lookout on the bridge yelled in that something was breaking the water

about a half a mile off our bow and all hell broke lose. General quarters was called on all

ships and sirens were wailing. Smoke screens were laid out. It was a Japanese sub. Two

of the big new destroyers went out of the convoy and we turned sharp with the convoy to

starboard away from the contact. This was 1300 time we heard a lot of depth charges

going off. There must have been 20 booms. We stayed on G.O. again for three more

hours. The new destroyers came back into the convoy two hours later. We don't know

what happened for sure but the rumor was that they sunk the Japanese sub.

We came into Dutch Harbor finally and we got into some calm waters. We had to tie up

along side a huge troop ship. We convoyed up and we loaded on fuel from them. They

carry four times more fuel capacity then we did. While we were tied up here came hats,

candy bars, army coats and all kinds of other things down our deck. Event ice cream tied

on a line handed on and the soldiers and marines were hollering on to us saying, you poor

guys are under water most of the time, all we can see are your masts. Boy, they yelled,

we feel for you guys. Now usually they put a big rope ladder down and our executive

officer goes to get further orders for us. We got to go up this time and when we do I

usually head for the ice cream fountain. Aboard the St Michael, a troop ship, they have a

regular ice cream parlor. I would run and buy me a big milkshake and I'd go out on deck in the sun. It was the first sun I'd seen in Alaska during the whole year. I sat on this big

hatch enjoying my milkshake and sailors are laying all over the hatch sunning themselves.

There were three or four sailors from the troop ship talking to a couple of our boys and

the guys were all looking my way. One of our men was pointing to me and then there was

some yelling. This sailor came running over and, my God, here was my cousin Jumbo

John Arabochia. We threw our arms around each other and both had tears we had to wipe

off. We sat and talked about our fishing trips to California for sardines in 1939. We were

on the Johnnie Boy sardine boat for six months. We had a great reunion and a lot of fun.

Chapter 10
New Rate, New Position

One year had gone by and we had been convoying troop ships on the Pacific Ocean for a

while. We have had encounters of all kinds. It was real exciting at times and real scary at

times. On our way home from Dutch Harbor I was told to take my exam for rate

coxswain. I kind of knew what was coming. Several times I had to take the captain over

to other ships in the captain gig, it was a 26 foot cabin like boat tiller with a stern engine

onboard. I had two rings on a kind dash board. I would have signals, one ding go ahead,

three pulls more speed, two pulls, stop and four pulls back up. Being that I ran fishing

boats of up to 60 feet and man boats up to twenty-five feet, I was good at landing and

taking off. At least the captain must have thought I was fairly good. That's how I got my

coxswain rating and now I was the captains gig skipper.

We were told upon entering Seattle that we were gonna unload all our ammunition at

Bangor Depot then head for Bremerton for some overhaul. I was again called to the

executive officer Mr. Dodd. I was told to pack my gear. Man oh man my heart was

pounding. I was sure I was being transferred off the ship. Mr. Dodd then said here your

orders; we are sending you and six seamen to gunnery school at Pacific Beach. Pacific

Beach was just a few miles from Ocean Shores. (I'm writing my book from there) He

handed me this packet and said you are in charge of the boys so get them together. The

bus, he said, will pick you up at 8 a.m. It will take you to gunnery school. It was

December 22, 1941 and I asked if there was any possible way to spend Christmas with

my mom. No way, he said, we are at war son. You are right in the middle of it. These are big guns you're gonna train on. You will probably end up on one. We will be in action

soon.

At 8:00 a.m. the bus picked us up in the Bremerton ship yard and we crossed the sound

on a ferry boat headed for Pacific Beach. We traveled for four hours. When we got to the

beach we had barracks all fenced in. In the small town there was a gas station, a

restaurant and a dozen houses. All we could see was a big bluff out in front of the

barracks. There were four big four inch guns mounted on the bluff facing the ocean. We

had lunch when we got there and got our bunks set up. After that we went to class and

there were about 30 of us sailors off of different ships. We got along real well and most

were gunners first mate ratings so we were odd balls, as they called us. On December 24th

we all watched a movie on the guns and how to operate them. It was interesting so the

day went by fast, but by the time night came we were all tired. It was Christmas Eve so

we all got a big dinner and by the time everything was finished it was 10 p.m. We went to

the bunk house. It was cold out and they told us it might frost by morning. There were

two bunk houses with 16 bunks in each house. It didn't take long for the trouble to start.

There were 7 of us in with nine other sailors from different ships. Most of the fellows

heard there was a tavern in town so some how a few cases of beer got smuggled in. It was

Christmas Eve so we had a few, after all our lives were on the line all the time and you

never knew what was going to happen. It could have been our last Christmas Eve. After

the cases were gone someone through a pillow at someone else and in fifteen minutes

there were pillows and feathers flying all over the place. The door suddenly opened and

here was our master at arms, a guy named Bull Hansen. He was the meanest, ugliest, 6 '4,

230 lb guy I had ever met in my entire career. He said, ok fellows you asked for it, now

you're going on patrol. The Japanese subs, he said, came up a few months ago and

blasted some of our shoreline. They may be landing on our beach any time, maybe

tonight, he said. But you will be there to meet them, so dress up warm and be out front of

the barracks in 30 minutes. Here it was Christmas Eve and freezing cold and we now had

to go out into the cold. So Bull gives us 45 Colts and we strap them to our hips. He hands

us a police dog on a leash and we went down steep steps to the beach. We had a small

flash light and a red light. He blinked the red light and out of no where in the dark

appears these four sailors from the school with dogs. Bull told them, you're relieved we

have some new recruits to do this. He showed us once what to do and we paired off. Two

of us went with one dog and we would walk silently on the beach for a mile. The dog

would stop when the two other fellows came toward us. You would have to blink your

light once and then watch for their blink back until you met each other. You would then

turn and head back the other direction. If the dog stops and gives a light growl you'd

better draw your forty-five and start praying, Bull had said. He didn't know it but I had

been praying way before I got to the beach. It was one of the worse Christmas Eves I'd

ever spent. We were about frozen four hours later. We were also hoping like hell the dog

didn't stop and growl. Finally we were relieved and got to our bunks. We had no pillows.

We were tired and I could have actually slept on the floor.

The next four days were all training on the big four inch guns. A target was close to a

mile off shore and we were to put holes through it. We changed positions on the guns a

lot and we had ear plugs on. After that was over I could still hear which surprised me.

Bull graded each of us and when we got ready to leave he gave me a big envelope to give

to Mr. Dodds or Mr. North, the gunnery officer. We headed back to Bremerton Naval

Base and I gave the packet to Mr. North. He took it and went into his barracks. Our ship was in dry dock at this point. There were a lot of rumors about exactly what they were doing to the Grand old Lady. One guy even said we were going to the South Pacific but that was just one of many rumors. Some of the rumors were scary too but we spent Jan 1st as well as New Year's Eve at Bremerton Navy yard. We got one bottle of beer with our meal which was a big deal. The next few weeks I was with three cousins who had just gotten into the war and were based in Bremerton.

My first cousin was a fighter. He was 6'2, 225 lbs, the heavy weight class. They had what we called smokers, Friday night fights, and he had sixteen knock outs out of sixteen fights. His name was Joseph Scrivanich.

My other cousins were Henery Zuvich and Walter Mezich. The three of us went through school together and when I had to leave I packed my gear with help from my cousins and it was sad good-byes all around. Where they ended up going to or what part of the war I don't know but they are all deceased today. I am the last of the three of us left.

I boarded our ship again and I saluted the flag on deck with the rest of the boys. I looked around the ship but I saw nothing new. No one knew where we were going or what we were going to do but we knew we were ready and maybe that's all we really needed.

Chapter 11
In Action and On Our Own

What was new was that they had added bunks in every corner of the whole ship. Forward to aft there were close to two hundred more bunks. I know we didn't need any more crew. We loaded up fresh food and, as with our last trip, we threw all the old groceries over the side. We now had fresh meat, food and supplies, we left Bremerton and went on straight to Bangor. We loaded our ammunition and then there was a big surprise, I noticed we took on a lot of extra groceries and two more cooks as well as two more African American fellows. One, his name was Jackson, was from the south. He believed in ghosts and was scared all the time. We became good friends. At least ten of the men aboard came to me and wanted me to go and try and find out what was up. A couple of our 1st Class Bosons also asked me to find out. We left Bangor and headed back toward Seattle. Now we were all really confused but shortly over the speaker came the voice of the captain.

"This is the captain," the voice said. "Will the 1st Class Boson mate and all chief's report to the bridge also bring Coxswain Budnick with you on the double?"

Oh boy, I thought, what now. I met Chief Mad Dog Barrett on the way to the bridge and as usual I was upset. But the chief said, Dom calm down, everything will be okay. I asked him but why me with all of you upper class men? He said you will find out in a couple of minutes. We all got to the bridge in a kind of circle standing at attention when Captain Vanness walked in and said at ease men. After we saluted he started to talk.

"Men we haven't got much time." he said. "We are going into Sandpoint. Look on our inner harbor charts, it looks impossible but the orders given are to go. It says to make sure to have bumpers put on the starboard and port sides. We are going through the government locks through the canal to this base at Sand Point. We are going to pick up

200 special troops, marines that are from the 2nd Infantry Division and get them up north

in five days. That means full speed ahead."

He told the chiefs he wanted to load up the troops, set them up and show them around the

ship. He wanted them shown what not to touch so they would keep from blowing us out

of the water. He told the Boson mates to get up in whatever lockers they had and find

fenders. He said to get them over the side.

"We have one chance through the lock," he said. "Now you, Mr. Budnick, do you know

where this base in Lake Washington is?"

He asked me if the locks would take us though okay and asked me what I thought. I

replied, "Yes sir I've gone through the locks at least 500 times and up through Lake

Washington many times." I told him that I had been to Sand Point. He asked me if we

could make it and I said it will be a very tight squeeze in some places but we could

probably get through. The captain said damn it why couldn't they load them on buses and

could have easily picked them up at Pier 91. These orders came from the Admiral Nimitz

so it was important. He said dismissed men, go on and get your jobs done quickly. He

added Mr. Budnick, would you stand by on the bridge? We may need your assistance. I

said yes sir. I felt like a big shot and I did come in use on the bridge. When we got a few

miles out the captain was looking towards the docks and said it looks like a dead end up

ahead. I said it is. I told him sir I wanted to let you know that there is a rail road trestle

and it's usually down. When we go through we have to blow three blasts on our whistle

for them to open and usually we have to wait for it to open. A vessel this size cannot stay

in as narrow a slot as it is so I advised them to have it up. Also the big locks have to be open we are too big and long to wait. The captain said they know we are coming and I

said sir I know the radio call letters to the locks, we talk with them all the time. What do

you suggest at this time?

Mr. Dodd, the executive officer suggested we slow down and I go to the radio shack and

get the radio man Grimes to contact them and make sure all is ready. The captain said,

good idea, Mr. Budnick go to Mr. Grimes and give him all the information and have him

call. Yes I said and I go to the radio shack and Mr. Grimes got the right channel. It took

him a while as that our radio aboard this ship was as big as the whole pilot house on the

fishing boat. We contacted the locks and they said they had seen us coming. They said

the bridge was going up alright now. He threw in a little message to the lock master and

he told him Budnick was on the bridge from the fishing boat the Debra Ann. The lock

master said you've see the boat go through often enough.

So I am on the bridge and we are approaching the big locks. The captain is on the speaker

and all the crew is at attention. I see from the bridge that they are trying to throw lines on

our big hawsers. Mr. Cullen who is now on deck is below me. I yelled down and told him

the lock people threw lines down and we needed to tie them quick. I explained that the

lock masters pull the lines and cleat them so we can squeeze in the big locks. I told the

men to get all tied up and stand by. The big hawsers lines are huge. I got in a little trouble

with Mr. Cullen. He came up to the bridge kind of mad. He said you're a coxswain you

don't yell at an officer and give him orders. I'm sorry I said, won't let it happen again. I

hope it won't he says.

We finally get through the locks and go through some narrow canals and make it to Sand

Point. We pick up the marines and we get back to the big locks. All went well. We cleared the canal and finally we were out in open water. I heard the captain say I hope we

don't ever have to go through anything like that again as he passed me on the wheel. In a

little over a whisper he said thank you Coxswain Budnick for your help. I said back at ya

sir.

So where were we going? We were going twenty-eight knots straight for five days with a

destination of Sitka, Alaska. I had been there and for this ship to get into Sitka, Alaska

isn't gonna be much different than going into Sand Point. Nothing much happened on

this trip though. These special troops were trained in 80 degree temperature and now they

will train in 20 below temps. That's a big difference.

It was getting up to March 1942 and for the next four months we convoyed troop ships

from Seattle to different ports in Alaska. At this point in time the Japanese had taken over

all the islands in the Rat Island chain. June 1942 was the high point for the Japanese.

They had four carriers, the Zuikaku, Zuiho, Ryuuo and the Junyo. The head of this fleet

was Admiral Hosogaya. Admiral Nimitz ordered our submarines up, one of our subs was

The Triton. Three days after my birthday on July 5th The Triton sunk the first Japanese

destroyer, the Nenohi off Agattu. There were only 20 survivors who endured the cold and

were rescued. On the same day our submarine the Growler sank the second destroyer the

Arare while two more Japanese destroyers the Kasumi and the Shiranuh were both badly

damaged and fled back to Japan.

Chapter 12
Operation Sand Trap – The Battles of the Bloody Aleutian

By now we were in Bangor loading on with ammunition and we were heading out to sea. We met up with several new destroyers and four Corvettes. We headed out southwest that was different than we had headed through the war so far. I was on the wheel again. We were headed south for the South pacific. We were going thirty knots and we traveled for several days. We then came upon the biggest fleet of big ships we had ever seen. We were fifteen hundred miles from Seattle and fifteen hundred miles from Hawaii when we met Admiral Nimitz' fleet, the battlewagons "Nevada", Pennsylvania, the cruisers San Francisco and Salt Lake City, the light cruiser Richmond and several more destroyers. We were headed north then to clean the Japanese out of the Aleutians. We were going to do our zig zag and the weather was rough, 70-80 mph winds, snow and ice. What a trip that was! Collins, my friend, was real sick so I took his place on the wheel. It was a real bad trip, one of the worse I'd been on.

The next watch was Tex from Texas. He was real sick too, as you can tell a lot of the guys were. There were guys hanging over the side of the ship and Chauncey all of the sudden yelled "man overboard". There were a few life rings dumped over the side but no ships stopped. No way were we going to stop when we were in Japanese territory. We were in sub waters. We ended up losing a cook at sea. A man wouldn't have lasted more than 10-15 minutes in that cold water. I said a few Hail Mary's for him. I felt bad since I was in with the cooks. I had an electric stove in my cabin and I got a lot of bacon, eggs, and ham from them. There were a lot of bacon and egg sandwiches made in my cabin in the gunnery shack.

One day later at 6 a.m. in the morning we got G.O. sirens. They were going off so we were running for our guns when Seaman Hurely was yelling where is the preacher Woodword. I stopped him and asked him what was wrong. He said he had a rip in his life jacket and wanted to find Woodword. Woodword preached to us more than once and had said that if we ever were sunk he had enough faith that he could walk on water. So Hurely says to me, I want to trade life jackets with him. He don't need one, he can walk on water.

We about froze that morning. A couple of our fast destroyers went after the Japanese sub and we heard some depth charges boom out. We had to be on double alert and watch for torpedoes. In rough seas they skip on the water and you may get to spot one coming. It was a very bad trip. Our rigging was getting iced up and it made it twice as big. We were getting heavy with ice in fact. One of the cooks who were left was named Clapp. He wanted to spray hot water on the rigging which was real funny. It wouldn't have done any good. (Clapp is still alive today. He lives in Port Angeles.)

We did have steam hoses and we got them out. We were trying to hold on to the steam hoses with one hand and our guns and depth charges in the other. We were losing ground real fast. I had had some rough trips fishing in northern waters but when I was at the wheel that day you could see waves as big as five stories high coming at you. The bow would go down and all you could see was ocean, no deck. How that ship didn't crack in half, I don't know. To this day I couldn't tell you what kept it together.

We finally arrived out about 200 miles off Dutch Harbor when we got orders to turn about. Four of the destroyers headed back to Seattle. The battle was to begin and the Japanese had carriers, battle wagons and cruisers. Later we learned that there was a good sea battle going on and the Japanese backed off after a few of their ships were destroyed.

They lost half of their fighter planes from their carriers. We heard that one ship of ours

ended up a real hero in that fight. The old cruiser Salt Lake City really tore into the

Japanese fleet and raised hell with them. It was then that were heard that in April we were

going to clean Adak out. We headed back to Seattle for now though. Our stanchions were

all bent back and so we were in Bremerton again for 7 days. It was a fast job.

We had to load up with ammo and supplies at Pier 91. We picked up one hundred and

twenty Seabees and we had to catch up with the convoy that had already left ten hours

before us so we had to do thirty knots. The convoy was doing only thirteen and they had

two liberty ships with troops that couldn't go even thirteen knots. We caught up to them

on the second day. We joined the convoy and it was another rough trip. We got off Adak

and we had taken it back over and brought the Seabees in. The Seabees were to build an

airbase. One ship in the convoy had these grading machines and a full load of the

Seabees. They made a field for planes to land on and it was just about an impossible job.

It was 25 degrees below zero with winds up to 70 knots. I heard later that up to one

hundred soldiers of our committed suicide. Another twenty-five were taken off the island

in strait jackets. That was how bad the country is up there.

After that we were called to Dutch Harbor which was quite a big base by now. There

must have been 50 thousand soldiers jammed up waiting for the big day. Amichita, Kiska

and Attu were yet to go so we picked up fifty radios and technicians and we were to take

them ashore at Atchirnoffky Bay. There was a sheep farmer in the bay only he and his

wife, so we loaded all this equipment and men up and headed out. We got close to the

bay when the captain made an announcement over the speaker. He needed two volunteers for a special duty. He added, Coxwain Budnick and 1st Class Signalman Aines report to

the bridge. I figured I would have to take Mr. Dodd to the beach but I got to the bridge

and he had Boson 1st Class Vanswaringer, Chief Boson Garrett, and our ships carpenter,

our Chief Machinist Johnson and us all lined up. He began by saying that this was a

volunteer job. He told us we could refuse if we wanted to. About his time I was praying

to myself. What now, I was thinking, why me?

"Men," he said, "this is a suicide trip. No one has to go but the top signalman Aines and

Budnick, I would like you to run the whale boat."

The whale boat is a twenty-six foot long open boat tiller with a stern and no cabin. It is

what we call an open boat. The captain explained that the Seabees had been in the bay

and had put up a few pilings and part of a dock that was put up well enough for us to

moor to it. He figured it would take us six hours to get in and out of the bay but we were

only 200 miles from the Japanese fleet and they had submarines out there roaming

around. He explained that the plan was to launch the whale boat at the mouth of the bay.

He said we were going to lash four depth charges, two port and two starboard side. There

would be two volunteer men with axes and the signalman. The signalman would have

binoculars and would have to watch the ship. The ship would have sonar sound on alert.

Budnick, he said, would patrol back and forth at the mouth of the bay. If while the ship

was moored up and unloading it got a contact on a sub, the two men with axes would get

ready and when signaled cut or chop the lines holding the depth charges letting them go.

The charges were set for fifty feet so and the boat, he said, would not be fast enough to

get away before the depth charges went off. So Seaman Challmer Clark, Seaman

Chauncey, who was a very funny man and a good friend were the volunteer axe men. We dressed up real warm and had a quick meal before we got into the whale boat. There were

a lot of good-byes and fellows it's been nice knowing you. There was also a lot of joking

as they lowered us down. We were turned loose and we gave a final wave good-bye. We

were kind of joking with each other but I was also doing some fast praying. I was plenty

scared. Aines had his glasses on the ship every second. I came up with a good scenario, I

said, you know this area is known as whale country and I wonder what will happen if

they pick up a whale on the sound and we have to cut the lines. Seaman Clark said I

wonder how high we would go. I said about fifty feet and that's whale boat and all.

Chauncy spoke up and said this whale boat would be kindling, there would be nothing

left of it or us. Signalman Aines spoke up and said we should get a medal of some kind

for duty like this and Chauncey said that Preacher Woodword should have been out there.

We all laughed.

That was the longest 5 ½ hours I have ever spent on the sea. I said many prayers I'll tell

you. We were a very happy bunch of guys when Signalman Aines said that they were out

heir way out. They were only about 400 yards in from us so all I said was boy I hope they

hurry out here. It's time for a whale to show up. I tell you there were six of us that

couldn't get aboard that ship fast enough. We got aboard and Chief Boson Garrett says to

me and Chauncey Clark that there were some rates for us. That meant I would go up t

Boson mate 2nd class.

We went to Dutch Harbor and ran two trips convoying marines to Adak. We must have

moved 10,000 to 12,000 service men to Adak. We were out of fuel so we were told to

fuel up and then meet up with a big carrier. We were to transfer a crew man over to the

carrier sickbay. He needed surgery. We watched as she (the carrier) came closer and

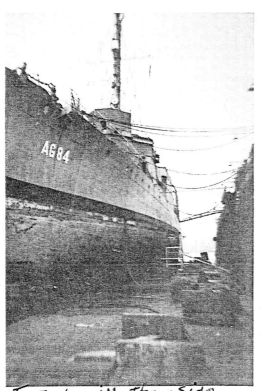

Torpedo - IN - The - Side.

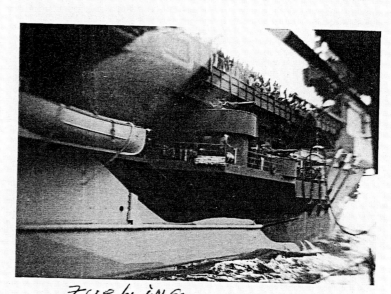

Fuehing

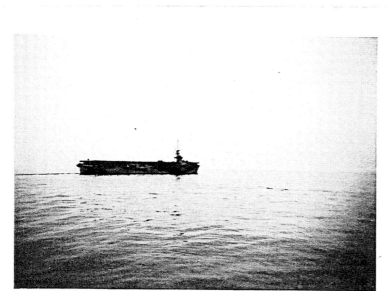

Pick - up - Woonded.

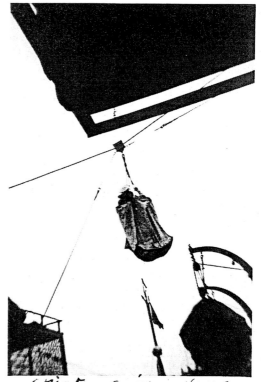

Chief - Going - Home.

closer. We got along side about forty feet apart and lines were thrown. Fuel lines were

stretched across to us. As we took on fuel we got a basket shipped to our bridge and we

put our man in it and he was hauled aboard the carrier. The fuel was finished and we

were back and ready for action, waiting for orders. While we were fueling there were

three big class destroyers in the area. They were circling around us to protect us. It was

quite a sight.

We had taken Adak and an airfield was being built. We got word that the Japanese were

trying to take over Shemiya so we headed toward the island to stop the Japanese. What a

site there was, Old Salt Lake City, the Cruiser, San Francisco, the battle wagon Nevada

and many more ships and destroyers were part of this battle. This made me get goose

pimples. To see such an armada! We were on general quarters most of the 24 hours we

cruised on the outside of our big ships. The big ships were in the middle. We got orders

to man our guns and get ready for the action. The Japanese forces were straight ahead.

We were to pull back and let the big guns in front. With binoculars all I could see were

blurs just like shadows miles away. Then the big guns started firing and man what a

sight! We could not use our four inch guns. They would not reach the Japanese ships. But

after about two hours of heavy firing there was no firing back at us and we got the

message from the Salt Lake cruiser that the Japanese force had turned tail and run. We

followed for eight hours, on go the whole time. Then the Japanese decided to head to

Kiska to reinforce their troops. Instead of following them we got orders to head for Dutch

Harbor. We picked up a convoy of 2000 men. We took them on a convoy of three liberty

ships of marines and landed on Shemiya. We had the Japanese surrounded now. We went

back to Dutch Harbor with the three troop ships and loaded them up. In three days we were coming into Amitchitka and our big ships were over there too. The marines went in

and took over Amichtika.

We now had Adak, Amitchika and Shemiya all within 250 miles from Kiska and Attu.

We understood the Japanese were bringing in more troops who were to fight to the death.

It was now October of 1949 and the weather was cold and wet, it was real bad. The

Japanese had no airfields finished and we were patrolling off Adak Island for submarines.

We were on alert at all times and now our bombers would pass over us and we would

count them as they were overhead. They were heading for Kiska and Attu dropping

bombs there on them. They came back over us and we would always count one or two

short. It was very sad to watch how many were killed. They (the pilots) were told not to

bail out since the pilots of our first planes downed survived only to be tortured and

eventually killed. It was a sad time for all of us who were there.

Chapter 13
Battle of Attu
Grand Old Lady in Action

There was a United States fleet near Atka Island and our ships were off Adak. We were

patrolling when we got contact on a Japanese submarine. All hell broke loose and four of

the destroyer went after it but the submarine shot her torpedoes and hit our seaplane

tender Caco damaging her. It didn't sink but five sailors were killed. The Grand Old Lady

(the Hatfield) went into action. Our planes dropped bombs on the submarine and we

started dropping depth charges on it with our destroyers. We weren't on top of that sub

and we damaged her but we were out of depth charges quickly. The destroyer Reid

finally sunk the submarine and five Japanese were rescued and taken to Dutch Harbor for

interrogation.

We were out of ammo and fuel after that battle so we headed for Seattle to pick up more

ammunition, marines and fuel. The big days were coming and we needed to be prepared.

Soon we were streaming back north but while we had been in Seattle the South Pacific

fleet needed Boson mates 1st Class. I was called to Mr. Dodd's cabin and was asked if I

wanted to be rated to 1st Class Boson and go to the P.T. John F. Kennedy's PT Fleet. I

said I would stay with my old ship and crew here. He said he was glad I'd stay. My good

friend Kleffener wanted to go so they upped him from 2nd Class to Boson 1st Class. I

helped him pack and he gave me his special dress uniform. It was tailor made. It was a

sad good-bye. He left and I got two letters from him later on. Three months later I got a

letter from his sister saying that his PT boat had been sunk and he had been killed. That

was another in a long line of sad days for me.

We took more troops to Adak and also took pilots into Shemiya. We had airbases in

Dutch Harbor, Adak and Shemiya. The bombers were bombing a lot from the last few

months of 1942 until the spring of 1943. The weather was freezing cold, 25-30 degrees

below zero. I spent a lot of time on the wheel watch. We were patrolling out in front of

Adak and Sheniya just off the islands. We contacted a dozen submarines in three to four

months. We dropped depth charges all over the place. We figured we must have sunk at

least three or four subs. Oil and debris would float up and that's when we knew we had

gotten them. We were at least sure we had gotten a few. The bombers were going every

few days and some were not coming back. It was a terrible winter with 50-90 mph winds,

snow and cold. That was why the soldiers there were committing suicide on the barren,

frozen islands. There was nothing there just tundra with ice underneath.

Some of the troops we took back to Dutch Harbor which wasn't much better but at least

they got to see an old movie or have a few beers at the local friendly tavern. On Adak and

Shemiya, Chirnokey Bay all they did was try and keep from freezing to death and eat and

sleep for months. They would try and work on the bombers and keep them flying. It was

the one place that many of the troops would have chosen the South Pacific or Europe

rather than be there. Anything would have been better than what they had endured there.

Many of the troops said they would never come back to this country if they lived. They

never wanted to see it again. Quite of few other soldiers went out of there in straight

jackets. I saw a few them go. This war in the Aleutians was a lot worse than people really

know about or ever heard about.

It was now getting to be mid-winter and we were a part of the Nimitz fleet. It was

January 12, 1943 and we had a new naval commander, Vice Admiral Thomas Kinkaid.

He came north from the war in the South Pacific. He brought the big carriers the USS

Hornet and the USS Nashville. The Grand Old Lady was really with some high class

ships now. We felt like we were big time. We patrolled out toward Kiska and just 50

miles at times toward Attu. Records show we caught on February 18, 1942 and ran into a

Japanese convoy headed for Attu and our ships including our ship opened fire with our 4

inch guns. Just within the past few months I had been put on gun number 1, it was the

gun on the bow of the ship. My job again was a suicide mission on that gun. I was glad

we had gotten our training in Pacific Beach a few years back. It really helped me on the

big guns. A 1st Class gunners mate would fire the gun and then there was a trainer who

sat on the starboard side gun and a sighter on the port side. One gun was elevated and the

other swung the gun from side to side till they were both on target. This third man opened

and closed the breech and the fourth man was me. I was handed this shell and the breech

would open ad I would shove the shell into the gun. When it was all ready the gunners

mate fired. I had long asbestos gloves on and if the shell did not fire they would yell

"dud" and everybody would leave the red hot gun and run to the opposite side of the bow.

The gunners mate would open the breech and the red hot shell would fly out into my

arms. I would run to the side of the ship and throw it overboard. There again I would be

praying a lot.

We shot off at least fifty rounds and one of there ships was hit and sunk. It was a cargo

vessel the Akagne Marv bound for the Attu.

The Japanese fleet fled with a couple of ships and made it to Kiska. The rest ran for home

when they saw that armada of ours with up to forty ships. What a sight.

We kept chasing subs and we saw our bombers going over to Kiska and Attu. They came

from the Shemya airfield, Dutch Harbor and the airfield at Adak. There were up to 100

planes over our heads. There would be one or two missing every days. That was not a

pretty sight. We had the Tokyo Rose. She was on the air every day telling us to surrender

or we were all going to die within a few days. She did say that an admiral Hosoguya's

with a heavy cruiser Nachi, and light cruisers Maya and Hiso, was on his way.

So with her warning our fleet was put on alert. We practically ate and slept next to our

guns. Then, in March, it came. It was cold about 20 degrees with heavy frost and 25 mph

winds and we got word that one of our planes had spotted the Japanese fleet ahead of us.

They outnumbered us. The Japanese fleet open fired first and it was 8:30 a.m. I just

finished my breakfast and I began to figure it would be my last. The Japanese let go about

10 torpedoes and their biggest ship, Captain Matsumoto Takegi's Maya, had our range.

Luckily we were in the rear. The first shells fell short and the torpedoes went by. A

couple of torpedoes just missed our cruiser, the Richmond. Then the battle got hot and all

we could do was let our torpedoes go. We let go our guns too even though they could not

reach them. We stood by and waited to fire at will and prayed. Man what a fleet!

The Japanese were over powering us and then about 9 a.m. the big old lady The Salt Lake

City, our big cruiser, with Captain Rodgers, opened up her big guns. It was 9:20 a.m.

when she hit the big Nachi. It was a hit on the bridge killing about one dozen Japanese

with about 20 more injured. It put their biggest ship out of commission and when we had

a few shells whizzed over our heads, that's when the Nachi was hit three more times. The

Richmond and all our ships were firing now and the cruiser Tama was hit and out of

commission. We were obsolete and our guns were too small and out of range to help. We were in the back of the fleet and now several miles away. We heard what was going on

over our radios. The Salt Lake City had gone right into battle and was hitting those

Japanese ships. But then, our main fighting ship, The Salt Lake City was hit 14 times and

our fleet had to turn tail and run. The Japanese fleet still had us two to one and they were

all headed towards us. All the destroyers, including us, got word to go and help. The Salt

Lake City was dead in the water so we opened the Old Lady up and put on our helmets.

We pulled the ammunition on deck and headed towards the Japanese fleet. There were

about ten of us destroyers and we came on the Salt Lake City. She wasn't able to move at

all. We lit smoke screens all around her and our destroyers let go all the torpedoes left

towards the Japanese fleet. We were standing by the Salt Lake City and it was now 1:50

p.m. The Salt Lake gave us word that she could travel but not fast. The Japanese fleet was

in sight by then and I said good-bye fellows, our orders were to stand by the Salt Lake

City no matter what. We were to stay even if it meant death. Then, it happened just like

in the movies. They were our heroes, B-25 Bombers going over us toward the Japanese

fleet. There were also 13 B-24's as well as the 11 B-25's. The Japanese turned and

headed for home. Those bombers save our lives and that's one of the reasons I am still

here today.

We took the Salt Lake City all the way home. We loaded up with ammunition and

torpedoes and headed back with our code name now Jack Boot. Admiral Kinkaid was our

leader and he led a task force of old battleships. The ships were, The Pennsylvania, the

Idaho and the USS Nevada. There were four heavy cruisers, one of our new carriers and I

counted twenty destroyers. We had four troop ships with over 12,000 men. We were with

World War I veteran ships with the Pennsylvania and the Nevada. We were all dressed for battle on May 12, 1943 and by 1 p.m. we had formed a huge circle. It made me think

of the old settlers rounding their wagons to fight off the Indians. At 1:30 p.m. we started

firing at Attu Island. Our guns were red hot and all the paint was peeling off the guns. I

dumped about seven or eight duds over the side. I handled over 300 shells. We fired off

for an hour and then our marines were loaded onto landing barges while about 200

bombers were dropping bombs on the island. Fighter planes were strafing the island as

well. The island of Attu is 38 miles long and twelve miles wide. It had rocky shores and

water that was ice cold. These troops were trained in the deserts of California and beach

waters where it had been warm. When these barges hit these beaches of rock the troops

jumped out and fell with full packs on their backs into holes four to five feet deep in ice

cold water. Quite a few of them drown before they got on land. I learned in later years

that one of my cousins never made the beach. He too had a full pack and dropped into

one of those holes and drown. In my opinion their training was bad. (Later in my story

I'll tell of what happened on this beach because not much has ever been told.)

Our troops went in there and we were not to fire on the beach. The Japanese were moving

inland and were waiting. The 7th Division went in there and it took two weeks to take

over Attu. It was called Massacre Beach from then on. The marines went in and the

Japanese were dug in on the side of a hill. They opened up on our troops and had our

boys trapped. They killed over 500 of our boys that day in a six hour period. Luckily

some of our troops landed on the other side of the hill and came down on the Japanese

from above.

Now while this was all going on we were on the outside chasing submarines. I'm sure we

sunk a couple considering what came up in the water. We had action on the outside and were alerted that the Japanese had a big fleet coming to protect Attu but when they saw

our fleet and that we had landed on Attu they headed back to Tokyo.

Around May 19th we had the island completely taken. We took close to 1900 casualties

on the island and we had killed about 5000 Japanese. There were many more wounded.

We went near the shore of Massacre Beach and lowered the Captains gig. I was the

Captain of the gig and Chauncey was my deckhand. We took Mr. Dodds to the beach for

some orders. He needed to pick them up there. To this day even with all the suicide

details I took on; this was probably the worst part of the war in my memory during World

War II. There we were near the beach in kind of a small channel and we had to take our

poles and push our boys out of the way. Those faces of young husky guys face up in the

water, I'll never forget them. They never made it to the beach.

We got into the dock and Mr. Dodds left the boat so I wandered up the beach a few

hundred yards. I saw big trenches dug and bull dozers pushing bodies into the ditches.

Then they were covering them up.

I have commercial fished up north after being on this ship for four years and I have put in

62 years in Alaskan fishing passing right by Attu. Today you can see rows of white

crosses lined up the hill. The last time I went by the crosses weren't so white anymore but

there were still there. I get cold chills when I go by there. The memories of that day have

lasted my lifetime.

Chapter 14
The Take Over of Kiska

Author's Note:

The writing of this book is partially to show people what they have not seen on television or heard on the radio. This was my life aboard a fighting ship.

The weather is very bad. On our ship we spent half the day steam hosing ice off our guns and rigging. There is a terrible listing of the ship and we were like a submarine, mostly under water. The winds were hitting us at 50 – 60 mph twenty-four hours a day. In the crows nest it was pure torture. It was just plain miserable and you couldn't stay for over two hours at a time. I couldn't wait to get to the bridge and on the wheel. It was the only warm spot on the ship. We had just finished the battle of Attu ad it turned out to be a very bloody battle. There was no difference between that battle and the battles in the South Pacific. We were listening to our radio on June 12th to Tokyo Rose and the Japanese garrison on the Island of Kiska would fight to the last man. Our captain spoke over the speakers and says that this battle of Kiska will be a knock down drag out fight. We found ourselves along side an ammunition ship. The ammunition ship had ammunition of all kinds so we loaded up and fueled up as well to our full capacity. We convoyed troops and supply ships to Attu as we had heard rumors of the Japanese 5th fleet under Admiral Koga assembled a huge fleet of battle ships. They were rumored to be, the Musashi, the Longo and the Haruna as well as the carrier Zuikako, cruisers Shokaku, Susuya, Kumano, Agano and Oyodo. They also were supposed to have 11 destroyers all heading with troop ships to retake Attu. According to records from June 9th to 24th we were on alert and had contact with Japanese submarines. We stayed on G.O. and our preacher Woodworth was canvassing the ship with his bible. Still he says to me that he has enough faith to walk on

water so I would say to him when we get hit and go down I want to be near him so I can

hang on to him and he could walk us both to the beach. We dropped a lot of depth

charges in the month of June and in the Japanese history records they lost a sub 1-31, on

June 11th the 1-9 and 1-7. In the month of June we thought several times that we had

gotten a sub but with 6-8 destroyers all dropping depth charges who knew for sure. I still

figure today that we got at least 4 subs on our record if not more.

We were convoying near Shemmeya and we heard several subs were sunk there also in

June. We were bombing Kiska with B-24's and B-25's. They were coming over us every

day and we would count them in the morning. Coming back they were always one or two

short.

In the middle of July I had a nice cake baked by our cook Mr. Clapp for my birthday on

July 2nd. I was told that we were patrolling off Kiska at that point. Our fleet was off Attu

waiting for the 5th fleet of the Japanese to appear for a big sea battle. Later the fleet came

back off Kiska. It was about the last of July when they arrived. We heard later that the

Japanese spy planes flying overhead figured our fleet was not to be attacked, they knew

they'd lose.

Our B-25's and B-24's and our fighter planes off the Hornet and other carriers were in

the air so the Japanese 5th fleet ended up heading for the South Pacific instead. Good

riddance I thought.

We had over 10,000 Japanese troops on Kiska to take care of so we patrolled off Kiska so

the Japanese couldn't bring supplies in for their troops. Their, the Japanese, food and

ammunition was getting short so things were going in our favor. The historical records indicate that destroyers of the Japanese fleet go in and evacuate troops of Kiska but that wasn't the case. Our fleet was watching closely and was ready for action. Rear Admiral Kimiura Masatome was head of the destroyer fleet and figured he'd sneak in for a quick loading of troops and get out real quick. He would have 5,500 soldiers to load so on July 7, 1943 he was coming in and it was foggy. It had been foggy most of that week and he wanted six destroyers to get in and get the troops and get out. But quicker than he thought the fog was raising and he found himself face to face with the Nevada, Salt Lake City, Richmond and USS San Francisco. He turned tail and headed back home fast. The records show a diary later found on Kiska. The troops had left so fast all they took was what they wore and their guns. The diary was that of a Private Takashi who was waiting for their ships to come and evacuate the troops. It read:

I am waiting for our ships to come and evacuate us. It is unbearable day after day. Our troops here are going mad. Everyone on this terrible place are exhausted from the terrible bombing an strafing. Please we want out.

Now his story shows that submarines went in and evacuated the troops out. I will never forget that light foggy morning. I was on lookout on the starboard side bridge coming out of the direction of Kiska. A huge hospital ship pulled through until it was 300 yards away. With my binoculars I saw troops lined up on the rails with bandages on and at the time I stated to Ensign Mr. Cullen, boy our planes are really causing damage. But now I think that hospital ship probably had a few thousand troops below decks. The Japanese claim they got the troops out by submarines but if that were the case, we had sunk quite a few subs so they must have lost a lot of troops.

We left Dutch Harbor with two other destroyers to fuel up and take on supplies. That was

on July 28th and 29th. It was during this time that the Japanese made a high speed run into

Kiska harbor and in 55 minutes 5,200 men were loaded and gotten out of the harbor.

There were two destroyers upon our return and there was gun fire near the beach. One of

our destroyers caught a sub out of the water and opened fire on it. The sub captain ran the

sub on to the beach and it was rally damaged. The planes kept coming, the B-25's and B-

24's, and kept pounding Kiska to pieces. Our ship kept patrolling back and forth.

One morning when it was nice and clear we heard a report that came over the radio and it

said all barracks had been destroyed and that their was no more radio messages from

Kiska. There was also no more anti aircraft gun firing on our planes going on.

A few days later we all got the feeling that something big was coming up. We were on

alert and we were told to cruise toward Attu to assist any way possible. Our battle

wagons and cruisers as well as destroyers were all there. It was the last days of July and I

believe, by my diary, that all we heard was a sound like thunder somewhere up ahead of

us. There were over 1000 shots and we were only 90 miles from Kiska. But once again

under the fire of our ships the Japanese turned tail and ran back home.

On August 12th we were patrolling and the captain called us to general quarters. He told

us to put on our helmets and mount our guns. Daylight came and there was our whole

fleet. What a site. Once again the grand old lady was with the classy ships.

Now this part is not in any history book and has never been on television involving any

of the battles in the Aleutians but I was there so I can tell you it happened.

On August 13th we formed our circle and started firing at Kiska. All the battle wagons,

cruisers and destroyers were in on it. We had gotten orders from headquarters, which came from the USS Richmond. I believe that Admiral Kinkaid came up with this but I

don't know whose idea it was really. We were given orders to fire all our guns and

torpedoes. This was an early dawn run on August 14th. It was a suicide run. Our

ammunition bunkers were to be empty, every shell, and all the 22 millimeters were to be

all gone. Our 4' guns were fired so much all the paint had peeled off of them. We had

some good shells and I only counted three duds that morning that I had thrown over. So

now what were we to do?

I see the troop ships. We were loading the troops into barges. Now the captain said over

the load speakers, "Sailors aboard the USS Hatfield, we have orders to be a decoy. We

are to go into the harbor of Kiska and we are to draw fire from the beach. We are now an

obsolete ship! We are to keep cruising until we are fired on. There will be a destroyer a

ways back from us astern. They will pick up what is left of us. So dress well and put on

your life jackets and helmets. Lay flat on the decks. Do not rise up or do any other stunt.

We have until 8 a.m., 22 minutes, until we have to head in so God be with us all. Thank

you men, let's go!"

So 15 minutes later we were doing 5 knots toward the harbor of Kiska. The joking started

and most of the crew wanted the preacher, Seaman Woodward, by them but he was on a

gun aft somewhere. My crew was in the worse position. We were all cuddled laying on

our stomachs right behind and under the aft part of our 4' gun. I remember I had my

rosary in my hand and I said quite a few prayers. We all figured the first of the shells

would go to the bridge, then to the guns. We would be next. Seaman Chauncey was on

my left. I had a halibut fisherman named Bakke near me too. We always had fun with him. He had a big ring on his finger. He bragged all the time that he had $3500 insurance

on that ring. Back in 1941 that was a lot of money. Seaman Clark was on Bakke's right.

I was laying there next to Bakke and I happened to see his ring on his finger so I said

kind of loud so the other boys could hear, "Boy if you get hit I'm gonna take that ring off

your finger." He said, "right now you can't get it, my finger is swollen and I can't get it

off." I reached on my hip and took out my dagger that we all carried. I said I got this

ready and I'll cut your finger off in a minute. He said, you wouldn't and I said laughing,

I'd cut your hand off to get that ring. The other fellows laughed an they all said you have

to beat us to get that ring. All Bakke could say was boy I thought you guys were my

friends.

The gunners mate had his phone on and said the captain called down to ask how

everybody was. He answered him that we were okay. We got the next call from the

bridge and they said, on alert men, we are entering the harbor. Keep your heads down.

We are in, or will be in, rifle range soon. No big guns. We picked up a little speed and I

asked the boys around me, hey fellows just think how many eyes out there are looking at

us and probably saying them poor suckers. There was 40,000 troops ready to hit the

beach. The good Lord was with us, we made a quick circle in the middle of the bay and

there was no firing on us. We headed out kind of faster than we came in. As we went out

of the mouth of the bay a big new destroyer went in and swept along the shore. We heard

a big explosion and the destroyer had been hit with a mine in the stern. Five men were

killed on the destroyer. Boy talk about luck, the Japanese left mines along the shore and

many more explosive devices on the island before they left.

That beach killed about 100 of our landing troops. All that remained on the island of

Kiska were three dogs and so ended the Aleutian invasion by the Japanese. We had taken

the islands of Adak, Kiska, Attu and Shemeya. The Grand Old Lady was in on most o it.

We had, according to history on the USS Hatfield, had over one million miles of convoy

duty plus we got, or at least I did, four bars for the battle of the four islands that we had

been involved in. I believe we, our ship, should have gotten more recognition for all her

efforts but this was just the beginning for our ship and crew. We were very luckyat Kiska.

If the Japanese had been on the island our ship and crew probably would have been

history.

So we continued to convoy ships and troops mostly back to Seattle. They were Marines

who needed R & R. They all needed a good rest, they deserved it for being on those

desolate islands. One day on those islands was like one month so I shutter to think what a

year was like for them.

Chapter 15
The USS Hatfield Gets Damaged

All of the big ships were leaving the North Pacific. The Japanese had shifted all they had

to the South pacific. What they left up on the Aleutians were a few submarines that were

harassing us badly.

Since August 28th and the take over of Kiska we had been convoying troop ships to

Seattle, Dutch Harbor, Kiska, Kodiak and Attu, most all of the bases. We were told we

had the milk run. We ran troops all summer and on into the winter of 1945. The year of

1945 turned out to be a bad year for the Grand Old Lady. Her end was near and we didn't

know it.

Now that most of the big ships headed to the South Pacific, (January 1945), we had

orders to patrol the Aleutian Islands so we played cat and mouse with the Japanese

submarines. We were at general quarters almost every day. We would get contact, drop

our depth charges and we always figured we sunk a few. We used to see periscopes

several times a day. And talk about weather, I don't believe there is any weather in the

world as bad as that. We would have 25 below temperatures, seas at 25 ft and sea ice

covering the ship. The winds would reach 70 mph and on up to 100 mph. At times we

were underwater 75 percent of the time. We had to head toward Japan and we would hit

those warm winds that would thaw us out as well as the ship. In just a few hours of

finding the warm winds it would be 70 degrees. We would warm up only to head back

into the 25 below as if going through a wall.

We were fighting cold and patrolling and I actually spotted a periscope. I was on the starboard side of the bridge freezing cold and my eyes were watering from the cold when I thought maybe I saw like a porpoise breaking the water. I strained my eyes and looked through by big binoculars. You can see a good mile away and objects look big with those things. But I looked good and realized that it actually was a periscope. I was so excited I screamed into the phones that I had on and told the bridge what I saw. I yelled, periscope, starboard bow, range ½ mile. Officer North was on duty and he spotted it too. General quarters were sounded and we went into action heading wide-open toward the submarine. We were supposed to have been on top of it when we dropped one dozen charges on her. We got contact a couple of times that day and we saw a lot of oil on the water as well as some debris. When night fall came I was on the wheel and North said I knocked the ears off everybody in the bridge. The joke on board for the next few days was not to give me earphones, just let me yell and the whole ship could hear me.

Another day passed and the winter months were going by fast. We kept in contact with our supply ship and loaded up with depth charges and fuel and kept chasing subs. Every few days we would see one of our destroyers but it seemed we were alone most of the time. It was March and when I think back this was probably the worse month of the war for the Grand Old Lady.

We were playing cat and mouse with a sub and we chased it way beyond Attu toward Komandorksi Island. We were determined to get this sub. The captain had been on the bridge for 15 hours now the crew was standing by our guns when right ahead of us we got a periscope. It was sighted and the Grand Old Lady let out a stream of black smoke and the skipper gave the word to get the charges at 70 feet. He said we were going to sink this sub with all the charges we set. We had 24 depth charges on our stern plus we had 16

on the starboard side of the ship as well as 8 on the port side. They are called Y-guns. So

here we were right on top of the submarine. We were doing 28 knots and the charges

were set to go off at 70 feet. The order came and we let go of all the depth charges. Forty

depth charges went on the Y-guns and they all went at once. The 24 on our stern rolled

one by one and boy was there thunder for about ½ an hour. My ears were ringing but then

the worst happened, the Grand Old Lady was hit by our own depth charges. We were not

fast enough to get out of the way and we were badly damaged. Our steel plates buckled

and our seams were opened up. We had all the pumps going and we blew ourselves out of

the water. We were disabled and limped back to Dutch Harbor where we were spot

welded as much as could be done in order to get us back home where we were headed.

We had a new destroyer running with us. We could only do 15 knots. We would probably

fall apart if we opened her up so we limped toward Bremerton. We were a casualty of

war. The scuttlebutt and rumors were hot and heavy. Some of the men aboard were

saying the war was over for us and others were making bets on what would happen to us.

We were told that we would be in Bremerton for over two months. What would happen

to us, boy we were all worried. They might put us on ships for the South Pacific. Who

could guess what would happen to us. I felt sorry for the Grand Old Lady. They might

just have to decommission her and put her to rest, a well deserved rest I'd say. Two big

wars and she was really tired. She probably wanted to rest. I was pretty sad and worried

back then.

We reached Bremerton and the rumors were that we would get some leave. I had hoped

I'd get to see my mom. I couldn't wait to see her. We got in during the evening and the next morning we were all lined up on the forward deck. The captain and all our officers

came on deck and we were all at attention. The captain spoke up and said, at ease men.

My heart was pounding and I didn't know what was next. The captain started by saying,

"Men I am very proud of you all. You are a number one rated crew. If I could I would

take you with me aboard a new just built destroyer but the new ships have all different

guns and completely new equipment. To train you all would take to long. My new ship

will be going to the South Pacific and you men are going," he kind of stopped an grinned

and said, "to a well deserved 30 day leave." Boy, a cheer went up and you could hear it

all the way back to the Aleutians I'm sure. "Officer North will take over now," the

captain said. Officer North started by saying, pack your gear and do not leave anything

aboard. He said, you will have a barracks at the base here by 1 p.m. We were to be picked

up by bus and taken to the barracks. He added that there would be an office there and that

Mr. Dodds or he would be there to take care of our leave, and, he said, further orders. He

dismissed us but said, "Mr. Budnick you will report to Mr. Dodd's cabin."

I was at attention and I said yes sir. I went to Mr. Dodd's cabin and I said, "Sir I was told

to report to you." He said at ease Dom. Then he went on to explain, "Dom what we have

is that the fleet needs some men on PT boats. The way you handled the boats with us they

would want you." He went on to say, "They want divers back at training school too. This

is volunteer duty and if you want to transfer to either of these positions we will give you a

first class Boson mate rating. You don't have to give me your answer until tomorrow

when you get ready to go on leave."

I went and packed and we got to our barracks.

Our ship was finally done so we were moved to Pier 91. Pier 91 was at Garfield Street

under the Magnolia Bridge. That is, or rather was, the 13th Naval Station for years. We

tied up to the dock there for a few days. They were going to take the ship to Kodiak on a

test run to see if she was stable or ready for sea and battle. I had one month leave coming

so I was taking my leave when the ship was to leave. When it was tied up to Pier 91 I had

60 seamen working under me and we were chipping away. I had to get that deck all

painted by the next day when our ship was leaving. There were offices on the dock right

where our ship was tied up and they had about 50 girls working in them. During coffee

breaks and lunch they would come out in the sun on the dock and flirt with my boys or

really bother us. My Chief tells me if I don't get that deck painted by the time the ship

leaves I will lose my 30 days leave. So I get mad and go into the big office where the

girls were working and ask for the manager. This lady comes over and says what's the

problem and I tell her that her girls are bothering my crew and I'm going to lose 30 days

leave on account of them. I was mad and I told her to keep her girls away from my ship

until it leave. She said she would try. As I stormed out toward the door one girl, a cute

one stuck her tongue out at me and made a face. I ignored her and went back aboard the

ship. It was 2 p.m. and we were painting full speed. We had until 4 p.m., two hours and

we finally got it done. I left the ship for home at 5 p.m. I got cleaned up and put on my

best uniform. I headed for the Crystal Ballroom to do some dancing. It was Friday night

and I figured it was a good night for a girl and some fun. I needed a big change in my life

at that point.

I got to the dance hall and the music started. They were playing good old songs out of the

40's and all. The girls used to line up in a bunch and the boys would go over and ask them to dance. We new a few good dance moves back then. The girls would kind of wait

for the guys they liked to dance with them. I had a lot of girls wait for me to ask them but

there were only a few I chose. On this great night I walked around kind of eyeing the

girls over when low and behold who should be sitting there all dressed up but the girl

who had stuck her tongue out at me on the pier earlier that day. I asked her to dance and

she said yes. We got out on the dance floor and I asked her did she know who I was. She

said no and I said you are the girl who stuck her tongue out and made a face at me today

in your office. She said, oh you look a lot different tonight. She said she hadn't

recognized me. She said she was sorry about making the face at me.

Her name was May Jorgenson. She was a real good dancer and we got along so well that

night that we would get up first when the band went on stage. We would do the jitter bug

so fast and so good that the crowd would form around us in a circle and a few of the other

couples would clap when we stopped. We met and danced Friday, Saturday and Sunday

nights and I ended up dating her through the whole week. I fell madly in love and so did

she. For the whole 30 days we were together a lot. I had our old 1934 Pontiac and use to

pick her up and we went to dances all over town. We also had picnics and went to the

movies. We both really fell in love.

I turned down the diving school. I did it to go home and see my mom. As soon as I

knocked on the door and she answered I knew she was glad to see me. We hugged for a

long time. We had a good visit.

Our ship finally came back and I had to leave. I found out that our ship was not to go to

battle again. This was six months before the war ended. We were to patrol. We all were

taking classes and we didn't know why. We were learning things like towing targets and about torpedoes. We learned about how they travel and what to watch for. We got liberty

every other day. Our officers finally came to one of our meetings and we got the rest of

the story. The Grand Old Lady was damaged beyond repair and was not seaworthy.

She would not make it in the open sea but, he said, we would know what our duty was

going to be in a week. There was going to be a lot of transfers to other ships as the tired

Old Lady was gonna have a skeleton crew. It was a sad day to see some of our boys

leaving. Everyday one or two transferred and mostly the gunner's mates. My good friend

Randy who was a gunner on my 4'gun, he opened and closed the breech while I shoved

the shells in and out. We were together 3 ½ years through four battles and it was very sad

to see him go. A couple of Boson Chiefs left and now we were a small crew of 197 men

with 160 left. Every day I waited for my name to come up but, thank God, I was not

transferred.

It was becoming summer, May 1st or at least I believe it was about that date, and we were

told that a bus would pick us up again.

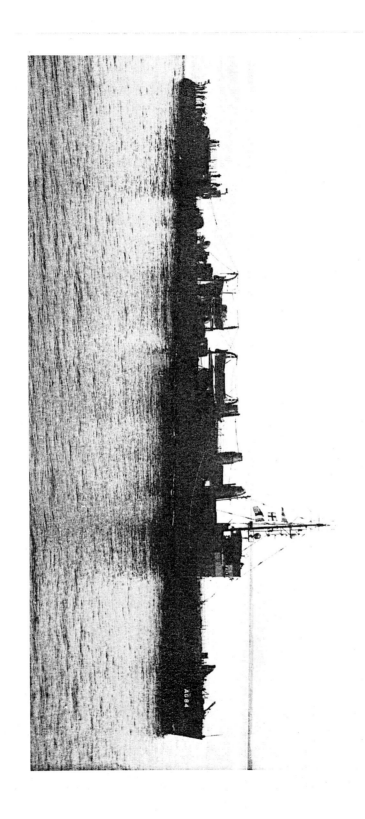

Chapter 16
A New Beginning and End

The bus picked us and after a 30 minute ride we were at the Bremerton Shipyard. Our

ship, or what was left of it, sat at the dock. She was a skeleton ship now.

When I saw the Grand Old Lady, a fighting ship stripped of all her guns, her DD231

changed to AG84, I got tears in my eyes. I know that, if it had been possible, when the

ship saw or felt us coming aboard she had to have tears too for the 150 men of the crew.

None of us said a word; we were a sad bunch of sailors. We had a winch on our stern

where our number 4, four inch gun was mounted. It was huge and it had about 500 yards

of heavy line wrapped on it. The mast was cut and half my crows nest was gone. All the

guns had just been painted up and down in the foreside. The foreside was all painted too.

My shack was all painted as well but later we did get fire arms, 45 rifles but that was it.

We loaded up with fuel at Pier 91 and I got to see my girlfriend on her job while we were

there. It felt funny not to be going to Bangor and loading up with ammunition. We were

finally out of the fighting war.

Our jobs now was to patrol from Port Angeles to Vancouver B.C. That is the mouth of

the San Juan De Funca straits. There was another ship called the "Eagle" and they

patrolled from 4 p.m.-8 a.m., all night long. We got the day patrol and left Port Angeles

at 8 a.m. We tied up at 4 p.m. and we did this seven days a week except when we were

out on patrol and we would get orders to tow targets for the ships. We did this about four

times a month and we also towed targets for submarines. Destroyers would fire torpedoes

that were duds. The duds were for training only. Being a veteran fighting ship we were given weekends off. The weekend constituted from 4 p.m. on Friday to 8 a.m. on

Monday.

I had the old Pontiac car at that point and would head for Seattle for the weekends to see

my girlfriend.

We would tow targets and patrol for the next three months. One morning we had to tow

targets for a destroyer. We had our target out 300 yards behind the Grand Old Lady's

stern. Our job was to spot the torpedo and mark if it hit the target or if it didn't how close

it had come. On this morning though three torpedoes were fired and two went toward the

target and one came right at us. It hit us a few feet below the water line and luckily for us

it hit out water tank. If it had hit us 6 feet aft of our tank it would have hit our broiler

room and with the pressure and crew in there it would have caused some deaths and

damage. Here we were in the water, no longer fighting wit a torpedo sticking out of our

port side. We limped back to the Bremerton Shipyard for another 10 day repair.

It was my birthday when we got back to the shipyard so I asked for 10 days leave while

the ship was getting repaired. The executive officer, now Mr. North, shook my hand and

said, "Boson mate Budnick if anyone deserves leave it is you."

I told him I was gonna get married and he congratulated me. I left right away.

I got married and moved to a housing project in Port Angeles. The rent was $12 a month

and there were a few married men living there at the time so my wife had a lot of

company. It was nice for the time.

The tired and beaten Grand Old Lady was repaired and soon we were back on patrol. For

the next month things went as fine as they could. Things were okay for once and there

were no major problems.

Now it was still war time and papa my grandfather was a strong Catholic. We were all

strong Catholics from my grandpa and grandma on down. I was born and baptized

Catholic and my children were born and baptized Catholic from the oldest to the

youngest. Before we got married it was understood by both me and May that we would

get married in her Lutheran church in Ballard because she had to take lessons in the

church from the priest. She had to do this for 6 months so we could get married. I didn't

want to wait because I loved her so much and being a warm blooded man naturally I

wanted May real bad. May, however, was a virgin and would not give herself to anyone

until her wedding night.

We got married and had a nice reception. We went on our honeymoon to Victoria B.C.

on the ferry. The ferry left Seattle at midnight and had staterooms. We arrived in Victoria

at 6 a.m. but did not have to get off the ferry until 10 a.m. We stayed in Victoria in the

Tower Room on top of the old Empress Hotel. It was like being in England at the time.

We had a nice time but we eventually had to come back to the war. I was sorry it was

over.

May had quit her job and we lived in a one bedroom house at the foot of the mountains in

the town of Port Angles. We got a dog and named him "Buffy" and a cat we named

"Fluffy. We lived very nicely for not much money. We lived on my $79 a month. We had

a lot of food from the ship I would bring home. We were very happy for the next six

months.

During the last of August one morning we woke up with the whistles blowing in the town

of Port Angeles. The town was wild and the speakers on our ship were booming out our

general quarter's sirens. The sirens were screaming that the war was over and Japan and

Germany had surrendered. We got back from patrol to the dock and it was full of people.

There must have been over 200 people all waving flags and cheering. We jumped on that

dock and got a lot of hugging, kissing and cheering. It was a big day for everyone, even

for the Grand Old Lady. She probably gave a sigh of relief, she could now rest. We had

to continue our patrol for another week before we got our orders to report to Pier 91 in

Seattle for further orders. My wife loaded up the old Pontiac and headed home to her

parents.

We arrived at Pier 91 and heard the ship was going all the way to New Jersey. The war

had ended and our ship was going to have to leave for the East coast. I was not happy

because that meant it would be another month before I could go home. In fact everybody

on the ship wanted out. We were supposed to get our according to seniority and the ship

was supposed to depart at 10 a.m. the next morning. At 3 p.m. that afternoon Mr. Dodds

called me on the speaker to report to his cabin. I got there and saluted, standing at

attention and he asked how I would like to get a discharge before we left the next day. I

said yes sir I would like very much to get out of here. He said pack your clothes and don't

say a word to anyone aboard. We leave at 10 a.m., he said, you throw your bag and

yourself on the dock and while we are backing out. You pick up your papers here at 9:30

a.m. I went around kind of telling some of the boys about how I was going to miss them

and I even told a few of them I was getting out. I went and told old Chief Garrett "Mad

dog" that I was leaving in the morning and he said, "You're a fine man, a good friend and

you will make it at whatever you do in the future." We gave each other a good hug and I

saw his eyes get pretty watery.

Morning came and I was packed. I had my last breakfast aboard the Grand Old Lady and

orders came over the speakers, single lines up. At 9:30 a.m. I went to Mr. North's cabin.

The captain was there, Mr. Cullen and Mr. Dodds. So you're leaving us, says he captain

and I said yes sir, but I'm leaving with a heavy heart. I'll miss this ship and the crew, I

said. The officers all started saying, you're a very fine seaman and friend and they said

that in fact I had shown them that you don't have to be an officer when you have

knowledge of the sea and a seaman ship. Knowledge, they said, like mine. Mr. Dodds

handed me a big brown envelope and said, "It's my honor to give you your discharge and

your four battle bars." He said he had hoped that I could have finished this trip with them

and that by the time we would have gotten to New Jersey I would have been a 1st Class

Boson. I smiled and we said our good-byes. The captain was the last to shake my hand

and said, "Boson Mate Budnick you have taught us a lot. You never once in four years

shirked your duty. You never refused an order and your stamina on extra watches and the

volunteer duties you undertook was amazing. You are the kind of man we will miss.

Good luck."

We looked at each other and the captain gave me a quick hug and left for the bridge to

depart. I went out on the deck and got my sea bag out onto the gangway. Most of the

crew was there. A few of the guys said good-bye. Clark, Chauncey, Collins, Tex and

Hurey, my buddies, as well as the cook Clapp, all gave me hugs. Buffalo Bill Cody, the

Preacher Woodworth, gave me his white sailor's hat. (I still have it hanging in my closet.)

My bag was taken onto the dock by Boson 1st Class Van Swearingen. He had been a good

friend for 4 years but he was the only one who was unhappy about the ship going to the

east coast. He said he had seniority.

I was there on the dock and there were 100 guys all yelling up all kinds of good-byes. I yelled back, hey somebody has to be on the docks to let the lines go. So as the Grand Old Lady backed out I stood on the dock and as the bridge passed by all the officers were out and I saluted and they all saluted back. I had tears in my eyes as I watched my home for four years sail out of my life. I watched on the dock until she was out of sight. With tears in my eyes and a heavy heart I found it very hard to see her go. We had spent four years together, fought those bloody battles, fought terrible weather and stood all those watches through the storms. After all that the Grand Old Lady sailed to New Jersey and then ended up in Washington DC. After World War I and World War II the DD3231 Hatfield was scrapped for metal. She finally got her rest.

Chapter 17
Life After the War

We moved in with May's mother and father in a little old house on 65th Avenue in Ballard. It wasn't long before May became pregnant and here came my very first child born in Maynard Hospital in downtown Seattle. It was a baby girl. She was a fat, pretty little girl so we named her Nancy May Budnick. We put a small bed in our crowded little bedroom. We were very thankful for that little room. Grandma slept in the room next to us. You opened the bedroom door and you walked out into Grandma's bedroom. Grandpa Jorgesen slept downstairs. He was paralyzed through half his body. He was a very nice man and told me a lot of stories about his travels in the oceans. He had been a towboat captain and had sailed many uncharted waters. I used to sit by his big chair where he sat all day and listen to his stories. He was a fine man.

Grandma Jorgensen was a smoker. Cigarettes were her hobby. She was a tough old lady with a kind heart who was a good cook and loved to see me eat. The more I ate the more she fed me. Soon, however, I found that I could not live with my in-laws. The baby was over fed. Whenever Nancy would cry Grandma was there to feed her. We had no control over our child, grandma would take over. That's were the trouble began. Nancy would wake up every night crying at about 1 a.m. and grandma would take her in her bed and play with her for 1 – 2 hours. She would smoke at the same time. Nancy got into the habit of crying every night until she was picked up. I wanted this to stop and big arguments ensued between me and grandma. I let the baby cry and cry; I even spanked her a few times. We could not sleep at night and grandma was always in our bedroom to take the baby. May and I would be arguing with grandma, the baby would be crying, it all got to be a real bad problem. I even locked our bedroom door and Nancy would cry for hours

until she was too tired to cry anymore and she would fall asleep. Grandma got so mad she

would not talk to us. She was getting very upset so I got mad one day and bought a house

clear on the opposite side of town. We moved to 10001 34th Ave SW. It was called

Roxbury Heights. The house was a nice two bedroom with a kitchen and front room. It

was a little war-time house way out at the end of 35th in West Seattle. I had a garage and

a big Oldsmobile. The car was black, 1939, with 4-doors. Old pop Sam Kampanoes gave

it to me for $300 and we got furniture from all over and moved into our very first home.

Nancy was 5 months old when we really got a shock. We weren't expecting it but May

was pregnant again. Another baby was coming. We were planning on five children but

not all within five years. It was too soon. My mom, who lived with my brothers Gus and

Mike, would come and help us by babysitting. She was real good with the kids and

helped us a lot. May's mom would come on the bus clear across town from Ballard. She

would come one time a month with shopping bags of food. She would bring hams and

meat and stay a day with us and then go back home. We loved her like my mom. May

was a good mother, money saver, cook and housekeeper. We lived real nice.

The winter of 1947 came and it was cold but I worked. I had gotten a job with the post

office and I delivered parcel post. Every job I've ever had I was a top worker. The post

office, at times, would hire 1000 or more people to help deliver packages in big army

trucks. They would load them up all night at the King Street station and we would come

to work at 7 a.m. and start delivering. Most of the guys would deliver a truck load in a 10

hour day but not old Dom. I had to be top, number one so I would empty a truck load by

noon or 1 p.m. and go in and load up again and go back out and be back in when all the lazy guys were coming in for the first time. When Christmas was over they kept me

working straight through. They gave me a Model A truck and told me to keep going all

winter which I did. I had a route of my own in town and I liked it and the post office liked

me. I delivered more packages a day on different routes than any other postman. I was

number one that winter. We had our first Christmas tree that year. The baby was strong

for 6 months old and I could hold her on my hand and lift her straight up in the air and

she would stay straight as a whip. The PI newspaper came out to our house and took

pictures of her doing her little trick. She was in the PI. She sure was a strong baby. She

was also pretty, she looked just like me, many people had said. She was a good kid once

we broke her of the habit of getting up at all hours of the night. She grew fast.

Summer came and I had to go fishing on the Col River and in Puget Sound. I needed to

try and make some money. I had another baby on coming and real soon we would need

more food and more clothes. As a dad I worried and I worked real hard. I fished on the

Hercules, a purse seining, in the Sound and made $1500. May had our number two child,

another cute little bundle of joy. They, the kids, were 13 months apart. That was real

close for kids but they were pretty babies and good kids. I remember coming home from

fishing and there was my mom at the door and she cried when she saw me. I came in

crying. May had just gotten home from the hospital and was still in bed. The baby was in

the crib and I looked at Cathy and cried. Me and Ma just hugged and cried with joy. She

was so pretty in bed holding Nancy and Cathy. Cathy was a good baby. She slept all the

time really well. She was pretty with blond hair and all. She was a doll and still is.

I finished fishing in the fall and had a few dollars. Christmas was coming so I thought I

would take a trip to Canada. Cathy was going on 5 months old and mother took care of

Nancy and Cathy so May and I went to Vancouver for a second honeymoon. We went for

four days and had a good time. We got home and it was cold.

The first of February we went back to work. I worked at the post office at the old King

Street station and I did so well at Christmas delivering mail that they kept me on again. I

would go to work at 8 a.m. and start delivering packages. I was parcel postman. I had a

route and all and I would get done with work at 4 p.m. then go to my second job picking

up mail from the big mailboxes from 5 p.m. - 8 p.m. I would get home after 9 p.m. eat my

dinner and got to bed. I worked Monday through Friday and had Saturday and Sunday to

spend time with my wife and kids and my poor mother. She stayed with us part of the

time and stayed with my brother Gus who lived near by the rest of the time. All was

going well. It seemed we were going to live happily ever after. We were in love the kids

were healthy but then May got real sick.

She had never been sick in her entire life but now it was February and everybody was

getting the flu and poor May seemed to have caught it real bad. She had a fever of 102 –

103. We went to our family doctor. He had been our family doctor since I was a kid; in

fact he had taken care of our whole family. My mother had worked for him as a house

maid in Interbay where he had his office and home. He liked Ma and all of us. He was a

good doctor. So Dr. Dillion looked at May and checked her over. He gave her some pills

but a few days later she still had a fever of 103. We went back and he gave her a shot of

penicillin, which had just come out at that time. She came home but still had the fever.

Once again we went back to the doctor. It was February 15, 1948 and disaster hit my life

once again. We got to the Stimpson Building where Dr. Dillion had his office and small

surgery. He took us in his office and said he was going to do some tests. He said it was a small surgery was going to be performed under May's armpit. They would check it out

and she would probably be okay to go home. Right after that he took her in with his nurse

and they did the surgery. I was waiting in the doctors' office. He came in and sat at his

desk. He got a small flask out of his drawer and a couple of jiggers and poured each of us

a shot of whiskey. He said Dom we took a gland out from under your wife's armpit and

its like a hard boiled egg yoke. When we took the gland out it fell to pieces. We knew

right way what she had. She has Hodgkin's disease. I asked, well what do you do for it?

He said, Dom, there's nothing we can do or that anybody can do for it. There is no cure.

She has, or the body had, he explained, 200 glands in it and May had an acute case where

every gland in her body is diseased. I said, well what happens now? He said Dom, your

wife has maybe 6 months at most to live. I told him he had to be kidding. I told him she

had never been to the doctor except to have the two kids. He said, I'm very sorry but

there is nothing we can do. I was so stunned that I told him I had to get some air. He said

May had to stay a couple of hours before she could leave so I tore out of the building. I

ran down the hills crying like a baby. I ran to the Pacific Marine Supply Company where

my brother had an office. I ran 6 blocks and burst into his office crying out of my head.

He got so scared, he asked me, what's wrong Dom, what happened? I tried to tell him but

I was crying so hard I was out of breath. (I remember that run today just like it was

yesterday) I told my brother, May is going to die. I told him what the doctor said. He said

are you sure, let me call and talk with him. So he did and he ended up like me, crying.

We were both a mess. He then told me to calm down and go back to May. He said the

doctor said it was best not to tell her. He said that if I told her she would just get worse.

He said that when got worse tell her they would have to operate on her and then she would be better. So that was the story and I got back to the doctors office and he told me

to relax and gave me a pill. I picked up May and we went home. I was telling her all the

way home that she was going to be okay. But the doctor told me I had to tell someone in

her family and someone in mine. So when we got home Ma was there and had us a nice

dinner waiting. The kids were all ready fed so we ate and May was worn out so she went

to bed and fell asleep. She would sweat all the time and she was wet with fever. There

was no pain but the fever was hot all the time.

After May went to sleep came the hard part. I sat my mother down and I told her. She

cried and cried. We were in our little dream house kitchen and it was 8 p.m. I had to call

Marion, May's oldest sister. I called and in between sobs and crying I told her. Marion is

the strongest woman I have ever met. She can handle any situation and not fall apart. She

is the rock of the whole family. She is a wonderful woman and a good friend as well as

my sister-in-law. So we were all going to have a meeting in the next few days to discuss

the problem and see what would be the best way to handle it. We met and we decided

that we were not going to tell May's mother and father. We were going to keep it from

them as long as we could so we would all act naturally. We were not going to upset May

in any way. So we started our miserable life. I worked two jobs and May had o take

radiation treatments two times a week. I would take her down and we told her this would

make her well so she was all for it. She and Ma got along like they were mother and

daughter. Ma loved May very much and treated her so.

May was taking lessons because she wanted to be baptized a catholic. She wanted to be

confirmed and receive the body and blood of Jesus Christ. She wanted to receive

communion so she studied real hard and went to lessons. Sometime in June she was to be baptized and receive sacraments. She was real excited about it. (I will explain further on

about miracles in the church and why papa is such a strong catholic and why May wanted

to be a catholic as well as the things that happened over the next few months of our

suffering.)

As I lived with May and we slept together and she had this terrible disease I could not

sleep at night. I did not know what was going to happen. I dreamt of funerals and coffins

and what to do. I dreamt of what was gonna happen. I was losing weight myself. It was

March and I kept waking up all night and reaching over and touching May. I was afraid

she might die and I would touch her and listen to make sure she was still breathing and

alive. I was getting so bad I had to get up some nights and sit in my front room and cry

until I'd fall asleep. I could not take much more. I finally took May to her treatment one

day and while she was there I went to see Dr. Dillion. I told him what I was going

through and asked him what would happen next and what should I do. He sat me down

and gave me one of his sample pills and told me what was going to happen. He said she

would quit eating, lose weight and finally one day she would get pneumonia. He said I

would have to rush her to the hospital. He said that it wouldn't happen for several

months. I was at least relieved at that. I was comforted by his words and help. I picked

May up and we talked all the way home about what she would like to do. She never had

traveled in her life. Canada was the first trip she had taken out of Washington. All she

wanted to do was to go to California and see the oranges grow. I called the doctor and he

called her radiation doctors and they said it was too late for her to travel anymore. She

was 97 lbs then and losing weight every day. It was just too late to take her but we could

take short car trips, 3 – 4 hour rides. Every weekend we would go to the mountains and where ever she wanted to go. We had fun. Ma watched the kids and we would go out on a

picnic when the weather was nice. Trouble was she got tired and would kind of doze off.

At home she would hug and play with Nancy and Cathy but she would get tired easily.

She was in bed by then a lot. I had to go to bed early so I could get up at 6 a.m. every

morning. I would have cereal and leave as Ma would get there to be with the kids and

clean the house. May would get up ad Ma would try and feed her but she had a lot of

trouble. It was at this point other trouble started too. Grandma Jorgensen always had the

whole family over on Sundays to dinner. Whoever wanted to come came and we went

most every Sunday but now the doctor was telling us, All of May's sisters and myself,

not to force May to eat. He said it would just make her sicker. And that she would get

upset and start to choke and vomit. He said just let her eat what she wanted to and that

was it. May's mom saw her daughter getting skinny and sick and as a mother she felt that

something was wrong. After a few times at Sunday dinner May's mom started to raise

heck with May and get mad practically stuffing food down her throat. May would get

very upset and we would leave right them and not ever finish dinner. Marion and her

sisters Vivien and Violet tried to tell their mom not to force her to eat but it was no use so

one Sunday we came to dinner and sat down to eat and Grandma Jorgensen just got mad.

She was trying to force May to eat and May cried, screamed and ran out to the car.

Vivien went with her and I blew my top so did Marion. She said we have to tell mom

today so I told Grandma Jorgensen the whole thing that May was dying and was not to be

force fed. She got mad and I got madder and we all blew up. We never came to dinner

anymore. Grandma Jorgensen came to our house and brought groceries and all but she

did not understand that May was really sick.

Now for a few miracles that May did. She was weak and could not go out on her own but she wanted to visit her sisters. Vivien lived in way out in Green Lake that was about 3 bus transfers away. I called home one day, as I did about three times every day, and Ma said May had left the house for a walk but hadn't come back and it had been a couple of hours. The neighbors' next door, nice people who helped us a lot, helped Ma and were real kind had looked for her but could not find her. I called Marion and she had talked to May and said that May had said she wanted to visit Vivien. Marion had told May that she was not strong enough yet but that they would come and visit her. So we called all over and no May. We called Vivien and Vivien said she was indeed there. She said she was doing some housework and heard a scratching on the door. She opened it and there was May, exhausted sitting on her deck against the door. How she got there to this day we don't know. She didn't know herself how she had gotten there but she remembered riding the bus. It would have taken at least three buses and she was on the road for two hours and ended up at Vivien's door. She did not know what number bus to take or how she had gotten there. I know now that she got there with the help of the Lord. Many small things happened in between these times. She kept saying when am I going to start to get better? I kept telling her she would get real bad and then get better. I told her she would have to go into the hospital before she would get better. I told her she would need an operation. It was a few weeks late when things got really miserable.

Marion rally was the rock of their family. May was the baby. She was eight years younger than the twins, Violet and Vivien. Marion had taken car of May when she was a little girl. The whole family was very close. They all visited regularly. Vivian was married to Harold Johnson, as fine a man as any man could be. He could do any kind of work and fix anything. He often helped anybody and folks could just call him for help and he would be there. He helped a lot and we have been good friends for years.

One night May woke up crying at 11:30 p.m. and said she wanted to visit her sister Marion's house. Marion's house was clean across town and it was 11:30 p.m. and we were all sleeping. May was determined and she cried saying she would drive herself. So I called Marion and told her what she said and Marion said to tell her we would bring her over in the morning but she cried no, no. She cried so that Marion talked to her but it did no good. So Marion said bring her here and you can sleep on the little day bed. So Ma stayed with the kids and said not to worry she would take care of them and we got all wrapped up to go. It was winter and cold out so we took off and got to Marion's. May dozed off at once and fell asleep. We could not figure it out. In the morning Carroll and I left for work at 7 a.m. and at 9 a.m. Carroll got a call from May who said that she found Marion in bed all blue and foaming from her mouth. She had called an ambulance and Carroll told her what hospital to take her to. They did and Marion had had a tubal pregnancy. That's what the doctor had told Carroll. The doctor also told him that in another 30 minutes her tubes would have bursts and shot poison into her system. She would have been dead in no time. If May had not been there, Marion would have died. I believe that when people are dying they know more than the living. It was all a bit scary but this was just one other thing that happened towards the end of her life.

Marion could not have children after that. May would always say she wished she could have some kids for her. I was always willing to help but I didn't know what to do. As it would come to pass, that phrase that May kept saying, I wish I could help Marion have children, she loves children, would end up happening.

May stopped eating all together. She had lost 103 lbs and was losing more every day. She was also now getting lumps on her arms and her back. All her glands were starting to swell and get sore. She was not in good shape. We kept her happy and I still dreamed of coffins and funerals. I had to keep it together because I had babies on my hands and my poor mother who was now not in good shape herself and getting very old. She was tired at her age and too tired to take care of May anymore. Poor Ma was suffering too. We just kept going and it was tough. May was still taking lessons and we said our prayers together every night. I would take her for walks around the block and rides up into the hills. She kept saying I hope I start getting well soon. It was the month of May and I had to put her in a wheel chair to take her for her treatments. It was hard, I used to take her to 5th Avenue to the Stimpson Building, park right on the corner and put her in the wheelchair and wheel her over to the corner drug store and she would wait while I parked the car and then came to get her. I would them take her to the elevator and to her treatments and then back to the drug store in the car and home again. She was so tired she would go to bed and sleep most of the time. All she would eat was ice cream bars. My children have one of the only fathers who make a habit of buying ice cream bars and eating 4-6 of them at one time. It is a habit now.

May got another one of her crying days and she wanted to live by her sister's house in Ballard. Marion lived on 70th and Jones so she wanted a home by Marion's so in order to grant her, her last wish we started looking around Marion's house for a new home. I didn't want to move but May insisted so we found an old house. It wasn't much but with a paint job on the inside it would do. This is where Harold Johnson came in. He was helpful to everybody and he helped me a lot. He was a good friend and brother-in-law. In order to get this house I needed money and I was broke. I sold my home but we got no money out of it. We hadn't had any money into it. The house had been like a rental and we had made payments on it but there was no money in it to get out. I ended up with no money at all to buy the old house near May's sister. Again my brother Gus came through and loaned me the $2500 for the first payment even though at that time this was a lot of money. Harold helped me and we painted the house and we were ready to move in. The big day came and we put a bed in for May down stairs in the front room and Ma and the kids were to sleep upstairs.

We moved early one morning. We had all our stuff in and I just had to bring May in and when I did she was very happy. We brought her into her new house and sat her on the bed and she began to cry. She blurted out that she wanted to get baptized now. I told her that it was in the planning stages and that it would be about a week. She went into a tantrum and said no, I want to be baptized a catholic today. So I called Father McGraph at St. Alphomsus and he said he would be right over. I told her and she calmed down right away. We cleaned her up a little, bathed her in her bed and she was an angel. She still had a few tears and asked where was the Father and when he would come. The Father came and I put out candles by her bed and prayed with her. We all prayed together. With the white sheets and the candles glowing I remember how beautiful she looked that day. Soon the baptismal was over and the Father blessed us all and left. May fell asleep in peace.

We went and cooked dinner. At 5 p.m. she didn't want to eat because the glands in her throat were so swollen up. She could not swallow anymore.

We all went to bed early but May wanted the girls in bed with her for a while. So Cathy

and Nancy laid by her and played with their mom. After a while she kissed them good-

night and we put them in their beds. May and I talked for a little and she said she sure

hoped she would get well soon or at least better so that she could play more with Nancy

and Cathy. I told her that we would all have fun soon.

On the same day that we moved at 2:30 a.m. May started to choke. She could not breathe

so I jumped up and called Dr. Dillion at his home. He said it was time to rush her to the

hospital. I called a medical ambulance and we rushed her to Providence. Once there they

out her in an oxygen tent. From 3:30 a.m.- 8 a.m. I sat by her bed while she was trying to

breathe. I kind of dozed off and on. I sat at the foot of her bed and I had my hands under

the blanket holding her feet because she said her feet were freezing. I told the nurse but

they didn't do anything about it. Finally, at 8:30 a.m. she called for me and I opened the

little flap on her tent. On the wall, facing her was the Blessed Virgin Mary. She said,

"look at her, isn't she beautiful. She is just glowing with beauty. She is very pretty." Then

May said, why she even smiled at me. She dozed off again and I told the nurse about her

legs being cold. The nurse checked her feet and legs. She propped her legs up and left. A

nun came in and looked at her and put a little medal on her gown. She pinned it on. The

nun, dressed all in white, held my hand and said Dominick your wife's feet and legs are

getting cold because she is dying. I cried. May heard me and she woke up and said hi.

She said her last words right then. She said, "I'm tired, I'm gonna go to sleep." And I

said, "yes sweetie, just rest, you will feel better." We were holding hands and she started

to gasp for breath, the nun pushed the button for the nurse and they came running but

May was not breathing anymore. The nun said she has gone to heaven. I lay next to her

and hugged her and kissed her. The nun took me away after a few moments.

We had a very nice funeral for May and she looked beautiful. All my relations were there

and we had a good visit. They all felt so sorry. May was only 22 years old and that's what

hurt. She was buried in Calvary Cemetery. It is a nice location overlooking the University

of Washington football stadium.

We tried to go on with out lives but then my mom got sick and having a really hard time

taking care of the house, the kids and me. She was cleaning, cooking and taking care of

the kids and me and getting worse. She was going on 50 years old. My brother Gus had a

small house with five kids. He was over loaded too. My brother, Mike's wife was sick

and under doctors' cares so I didn't know what to do. It seemed that there was just one

misery after another. There was no end to my suffering. We decided to look at

orphanages. We went to a place called Holy Angels out of town a ways. Ma and I went

looking but it was terrible. All the little babies were crying in their cribs and my girls

were so small, they would have had to stay in one of those cribs all day. Some of the

babies diapers hadn't been changed, it was bad. I could not stand it. We left there

knowing that we could not leave my girls there.

My brothers Mike and Gus heard I was looking to put the girls some place. They decided

that they were going to take one a piece and split the girls up. Gus was going to take

Nancy and Mike was going to take Cathy. Mike's wife wanted a girl really bad. It was at

this time that Marion heard I was having a hard time so she had us over to dinner. It was

then that she said she would be glad to take both girls until I got on my feet and paid my

bills. I owed $11,000 to doctors and radiation treatments. I had bills of all kinds. The situation with Marion worked out fine. I began fishing again and I went to Alaska. I was

gone from May until November and when I got home I was glad I could see my kids.

I lost my house. I lost it to a bunch of crooked real estate people. The filed for the house

and took it away from me. I left again for fishing in the south. By April I had made

enough money to pay off all my debts with the doctors and I even paid my brother Gus

back. I felt pretty good by then. It was good to be even again.

I was getting ready to go fishing in Alaska again but I visited the kids regularly when I

was home. Every weekend and even at times in the middle of the week I would pick them

up and take them for walks or go play with them. I was lonely though too. I used to walk

the streets looking for May. It seemed she was always in my vision. I sure missed her. I

cried a lot of nights and many nights fell asleep crying. I couldn't stay with the kids at

Marion's so I stayed at my brothers' house out in west Seattle. I slept in the basement.

Ma and me were making fishing net and talked about my problems while we did. Night

after night we would talk but I didn't know where to turn.

One day Marion and Carroll called me over to their house for dinner. After dinner I knew

something was up because of the way Marion and Carroll were acting. We sat down in

the living room in their little house. (Cathy lived there in later years too) Marion looked

at me and said, "Dom, we invited you over to have a very serious talk with you." She

said, "We know it will hurt you to even hear what we have to say but you remember how

you felt when May died. You remember how bad it all was for you? Do you remember

how bad you felt when she left? Well the children have been with us for a year now and

we love them like they were our own. We know though that their will come a day when

you will meet another girl and get married and come to take the girls. It would be like a death in our family for that to happen. It would be like killing us off to have to give these

girls up. We want to adopt the kids and raise them as our own. We will build a new house

next door to us here. We own the lot and we will have a bedroom for each girl. We would

clothe them and they would have all they needed for school and college. We will do all

this if we can have the children.' If not, she said, you will have to take them so we won't

get so close to them. It would really kill us when they had to leave and we can't handle

that. They wanted me to think about it for a bit and then call and tell them what I had

decided. As soon as I did they would start building on their new home.

I had had the feeling all evening that they were going to tell me that they couldn't take

care of my kids anymore. As it turned out I had a choice as to what to do. I talked it over

with my family and everyone said the same thing, what would I have to give the kids.

How would I take care of them? How would I raise them with no money and no home?

The other thing my family pointed out was that at least with Marion the girls would still

be in the family. Marion and Carroll had already told me that I could come over anytime I

wanted to and visit. When the girls got old enough to understand they would explain it to

them who their dad was and what had happened. So the decision was made and on the

next Sunday I went out to Marion and Carroll's house and told them what I had decided. I

told them they could adopt Nancy and Cathy. They just cried with joy as May and I had

when the girls had been born. May had always said she wished we could have had some

children for Marion and Carroll. It seemed the good Lord had this all planned out in His

book of what was to come.

We got an attorney, Stan Soderland who is a judge now but was just a young attorney

then when we first met, and he did all the paperwork for us. It all turned out perfectly.

Marion and Carroll were well off and they built a nice home. The girls' closets were

filled with pretty dresses and clothes. I could have never given those kids what they got

from Marion and Carroll. I was gone most of my life fishing. My kids I had later hardly

ever seen me. I would still come and visit though. I felt bad some times because the girls,

especially Nancy, would come and jump into my arms and not leave until I was ready to

go. Cathy, who was pretty young then, 6 months when her mom died, hung on Carroll. I

decided then that it was probably best that I didn't come around all the time even though

my heart was breaking. I wanted to cuddle the girls and play with them but I couldn't

because it hurt so much. I stayed away as much as possible. I needed to give Marion and

~~Harold~~ *Carroll* their home and let them give the girls the love they had for them. I stayed away as

the girls grew and they got to know me as Uncle Dom. I used to park on the street and

watch the girls walk home from school. I would sit and cry. I wanted to pick them up and

cuddle them and listen to them start to talk. I wanted to hear them learn to read and write

but it wasn't to be. I used to cry at night and wonder what they were doing. On those

nights I knew one thing, they were getting the best of care and they were eating well.

They had a nice loving home and that was what made me feel better.

At that point I lived in an old milk truck on pops station on 15th Ave. West just in the

town side of Ballard Bridge. (There's a car wash there now.)

Chapter 18
Another New Beginning

In 1949 my life was a mess and had, to some degree, ended. I was down a lot, I had no

wife, no children and as far as I was concerned, no life. I had no home and no furniture. I

felt like I was just in a real mess. I was walking the streets all the time looking for my

wife who had died. Things were hard. I was living with my brother Gus at that point and I

slept in the basement. Ma was there too as well as Gus and his kids. He was the dad in the

family and he took care of all of us. We were all stuck together.

I fished the Columbia River where I was born and I fished Puget Sound and alas I

considered myself a top fisherman. I worked hard and long hours in any kind of weather,

good or bad. I really suffered fishing the Columbia River, it was hard fishing and it made

for a tough miserable life. I was living in the little bow picker boats and moving in to old

houses trying to make a living. It really was a tough life.

My mother and I were living in the basement at my brother Gus' home when I wasn't out

fishing. We made fishing net together and it was all done by hand. It was a mesh net. We

had a lot of linen that Gus had brought home from Pacific Marine where he had been the

boss for 30 years. Week after week we sat in the basement on that net and we talked a lot.

Ma told me a lot of stories about her life and about my dad as well as different things that

happened in her life. That was the year I got to know my mother real well. She told me of

the miseries she had gone through in her life. I miss those talks.

Now I went fishing with Matt Svornich on the boat the Vernon. A friend of mine named

Bob Campion was on the boat. Bob was a fisherman, a sail maker and a teacher of

navigation. He was very smart and a good man. We fished all summer on the cape and all over. It was a very good summer for me since I had good company. They kept me going

and we had fun so the summer went by fast. Winter came and it was time for me to work

at Pacific Marine. We salvaged nets and I made leads for trolling boats for Cash, he was

my boss on the 4th floor with Gus. I also picked up mail for parcel post US Mail. I

worked all winter.

In January of 1949 I worked all winter trying to pay for my bills. I had had $11,000 in

doctor and hospital bills to pay so I had made arrangements to make payments. I worked

two jobs and fished the Columbia River in Brookfield in May. We went to Bristol Bay

but the best years were over now. I went with Gus and Svornich and we chartered a tuna

clipper form California and ten of us got two sailboats and my bow picker. On May 13

we loaded them all on the tuna clipper and boy what a safari that was. It turned out to be

a real thrilling experience that trip. We fished Bristol Bay and were gone for two months.

We had caught 33,000 fish so we headed home. I sold our fish and I took my boat and

went back to the river for august fishing. This turned out to be another suffering mess.

We lived in Brookfield and Ma was there as well as Gus and his family. We had the

family all together. My brother Mike had a punch board business east of the mountains be

he had to go and play baseball for another season. He wanted me to buy his route. It was

200 restaurants and taverns and went from Seattle all over eastern Washington and ended

up at Republic which was up in the mountains. It ended up being a real experience. I

would leave on a Monday morning in a 1948 panel Ford truck. That was a real go-er that

old truck, it never failed.

It was winter and it was one of the coldest winters east of the mountains in history. We

had days and nights of 40 degrees below zero. Several people died in the freezing weather. Some kids had died that year when a bus stalled in a snow bank. Before they

were found they had froze. It was a real cold, bad winter but I did meet a lot of nice

people. I would get up to Republic in a week and then head back through another part of

my route and get home Friday. After being gone two weeks I saw the Chief Joseph Dam

being built because it was one of my stops. It was different because it was a construction

camp. There were real nice people there though.

I also learned to tend bar and wash dishes in the restaurants. I learned to smoke cigars too

so I was getting up in the world. It was hard driving in the snow and freezing ice. The

streets and hills were scary at times. I plowed right through them. There would be 10 foot

high snow banks sometimes in Cle Elum and Ellensburg. I did not want to freeze to death

so I pushed on. When I got back to town I used to buy my boards and all from the stores

in town. Finally not knowing what was happening to me the owners put me out of

business. I worked a deal where I traded my route for a new 1950 Pontiac Streamliner V8

Straight 8. It was one of the best cars I owned.

Spring was coming again and I was going to go fishing again. It was April and time to

head for the Columbia River and Brookfield once again. I was living in an old van at

Sam's station in Interbay at the time as that Gus' house had gotten too crowded. We had

to do some thing. Ma fixed me a bed and came and cleaned that old van up for me. It was

real hot in the summer and real cold in the winter. Thanks to my good and best friend old

Sam Campanoes I had a place to live. He was a real Santa Claus. Papa Sam, as he was

known by everyone, had a big heart. He was like a dad in so many ways. I lived with him

at the station for years. I liked it in the van behind him. He gave me so much good advice

and he helped me through my troubles. By the way he nick name me "troubles" too. He'd say here comes troubles. He gave me cars to use and during the war and he gave me gas,

all I needed. We had to have stamps for gas and he gave me food too. He was a friend to

all who knew him. He was born on Christmas Eve and he died on Good Friday.

That fall went a long well and I visited the kids and the family. Every thing seemed to be

getting along well. I was getting my life back in order but I was starting to drink a little

and raise heck. I had a new car and was driving. I thought I was bad. I could tell some

unbelievable stories. I want my kids and grandkids to look up to me though so I won't tell

those. I want my grandkids to see grandpa as a hero. All my life I have had real good will

power. I could stop doing anything I wanted. I never drank too much and one day I quit

completely. I never smoked but a few cigars years ago and I never tasted or smoked any

dope. I lived a fairly healthy life but that was about to change.

I had lumps under my armpits, that's what the doctors called them, lumps. I went to my

doctor, Dr. Dillon and he said, "I have bad news for you, we took a biopsy of your tumors

under your armpits and they show cancer." He said they would have to operate at once. I

told him okay and the doctor operated on me. He took all my tumors out and it all turned

out okay. I had no way of knowing that this was the first cancer surgery of what would be

12 total. I got well this time though and within a few weeks I was out dancing and

enjoying myself.

Chapter 19
Steps Forward

I used to go to Parkers on Saturday nights. I had a friend named Florian and we called

him jiggalo. I met him at Parkers one Saturday night and he said he had a girlfriend

named Shirley with him. He said she had a girlfriend and wanted to know if I wanted to

meet her the next Saturday night there at Parkers. I said I'd take a look at her and that

yes, I would be there. So the next Saturday night, around the first Saturday in September,

I went to Parkers with my gang. There were about 15 of us and we started drinking. After

a short time here come Florian and he says he's got my blind date and that she was in the

bathroom if I wanted to meet her. I said I would take a look at her so we went to the

women's bathroom and out came my blind date. She had a dress on that went almost to

her ankles and she was the most beautiful girl in the ballroom that night. I was introduced

and we danced. She was okay but had a Missouri hop but I figured I could change that

style. She kept me about two feet away from her since I was drinking. She didn't drink.

So we danced the night way and the evening finally ended. I got to take her home, she

lived in Everett. The boys laughed at me as we took the girls that far away home. We

took off for Everett though, 30 miles from Seattle.

We got to her girlfriends house in Everett and got to the porch and said good-night but

not until I got at least a good-night kiss and that kiss was it. She always told me for 40

years that after she kissed me that night she knew I was the man for her. But the Budnick

kisses are fatal. One kiss and that's it, it is all it takes.

This was the first of September and I started dating steady every Wednesday. I'd take her

out on Saturday and Sunday. I made a lot of trips back and forth. She worked for a Dr.

Measer, a dentist in Cathlamet where I was born. Dr. Measer used to do our teeth when I

was young. The first year was amazing. We went all over town dancing and eating. I

knew I was in love again. After losing may I never thought I would ever be in love again

but the good Lord helps and he sure helped me. I needed it too because I was going down

the drain pretty fast and now I was happy and in love again.

I got to meet her parents and we all got along really well. She had a real nice family.

Dolores, that was her name, was also in love with me but I could never figure out why

she loved me. I had been married before and had two children and all. I was also eight

years older than her. But she loved me.

We went together for months and then Christmas came and I gave her a wedding doll. I

took her to the park and gave her the doll and told her to look at the pretty underclothes

the doll was wearing. When she looked there was a box under there. When she opened it

there was a nice diamond engagement ring. I asked her to marry me and she said yes. We

kissed and talked about getting married in February on a Saturday morning. By the time

we left the park it was set.

New Years came and went and we took her mom and dad to Parkers on New Years Eve.

The really had fun and could not believe the sights they saw out there.

The big wedding day came and we got married in the Monte Cristo Hotel in Everett. She

was talking lessons through the Catholic Church and became catholic. Our marriage was

blessed by the Father in the sanctity of the church. We then took a honeymoon trip and

spent one month in California. We visited her brother, step-mom Wandine and her real

dad Glenn Hermann. They were all real nice people. Her dad got us an apartment across

the hall from where they lived and took us all over. We went to Disneyland and Knots

Berry Farm. We even took one night and drove to Long Beach and went dancing in the

Treanon Ballroom. We danced to a band called Lawrence Welk. Who knew at that time

that he was going to become big? At that time he was an unknown band leader. Later he

had his own television show for many years. I have tapes for the VCR on his band.

So we went to Mexico and down to Tijuana. We went al over and I had my new Pontiac.

It really was the best car I had ever owned. (In all my years.)

We traveled all over California, to San Francisco, Oakland, the San Diego Zoo and

Anaheim Stadium. We saw a Los Angeles big league pro baseball game. Dolores' dad

was a very nice man. He treated me like a son. All of her family treated me well.

We enjoyed ourselves but it was finally time to head home. We stopped in Astoria,

Oregon and saw all my relations. I took my new bride to my home town of Brookfield

were I lived from birth until I was 9 years old.

We were taken there by my cousin John by boat and lived in a house with rats. We slept

in our clothes the first night since we had not cleaned up. We got up in the morning and

there was a foot of snow on the ground. It was really coming on and we were supposed to

leave in two days but no one came to pick us up. My cousin left us with some potatoes

and a big chunk of Salmon but that was it. We found a few cans of food in the old house

and we ate that up. Really soon though we were out of food.

There was a woman who lived one mile up in Jim Crow Creek. She was the mail lady

and the Gregets were the only other people in town. They brought us some onions and

food. My cousin finally made it after the big storm was over and picked us up. It had

been quite an experience.

We got home to Seattle and stayed with my brother Gus while we started looking for a

house. I had $4,400 in the bank, a new car and the clothes on my back. It was March

1951. Gus lived on the corner of Holden Street and 31st SW. We found a little shack of a

house for $5,000 up the street at 7521 31st SW. It was just 5 houses up from my brother

and my mom. Mom still lived with my brother most of the time.

So we got paint and painted the little house. I went up to Sears and bought all our

furniture and we started our new life together. We were really in love and had a nice

home for a start.

I had my first surgery about then. I had a hemorrhoid operation and had to take it easy for

a couple of months. I hung some nets in my back yard for Alaska and I drew

compensation for the first time in my life. It was also the last time in my life I ever got

anything for free. I drew $30 a month. We lived on $90 a month for lights, food, and

phone and all but we lived just fine. We made it good and had a nice beginning. I was

happily married again.

We went along until the May season and then we went to the Columbia River. I fished a

drift right I had and Delores came with me. We lived in the old house on the beach and

fished every year for 50 years. I fished the Columbia in the month of May and in August

and September as well as from October through November. From June 1st to July 30th I

would go to Alaska and Bristol Bay. It was the same routine I had for 56 years. I was in

Alaska for 62 of my birthdays. At one time I had three fishing boats and I kept them all in

good shape. I fished and worked in different jobs in the winter. I long shored a few

winters. I worked for the post office a few years but mostly I worked for Pacific Marine

Supply Company. We worked the nets for Alaska. My brother Gus was the supervisor for

Pac Marine for 36 years. He also fished a few seasons.

We lived nice, me and Dolores. For the next few years she fished with me in the

Columbia River and was a real good cook and housekeeper and lover. In 1953 our first

child was born, a beautiful baby girl we named Debbie. She was a pretty baby and I saw

her being born. That was one of the biggest thrills of my life. She was a doll and to this

day she still is. She was never a problem. She was a little lively as I always was.

Dolores was a good mother. Although she only wanted a couple of kids she was okay

with more. I already had a couple of girls and now a third but I also wanted a son. I

wanted someone to carry on the Budnick name. So we tried again and in 1955 I got my

wish and our prayers were answered with a baby boy. What a boy he was. We named him

Daniel Joseph Budnick. He was a little white haired husky little guy. He never cried at

night. In fact from the time he was born he never cried at night. He was a quite little boy.

He was a good boy though and as it turned out all his life he was husky. He is all of 225

lbs at 6' 2 and he has just as big a heart. He was a good worker too. He is 40 years old

today and often fishes with me on the Col River and Puget Sound. He fished for 12 years

with me in Alaska. He did a good job too, I was always proud of him as a son.

I worked for years at the same old routine. Every year I would start my year on May 1

and until the 30th I would fish the Col River. I would then come home to Seattle, get

packed and ready to leave for Bristol Bay where I would fish from June 15th – July 21st. I

would then come home and take a vacation with the kids for a few weeks. We went to

Disneyland in California, we went back east several times and to Missouri as well as all

over the state of Washington. Then August 15th would come and I'd go to the river again.

We lived for a while on an island called Woody Isle. My mother was born there and we

had a nice big home on the island. I had a lot of friends come and visit us there. We had

some real interesting stories about the place, so many I could write a book on the

experiences I had there.

In 1956 in Bristol Bay we went north on the ship "The North Star". It was the ship that

Admiral Byrd took to the artic ocean. It had quite a history. It was bought by Auggie

Mardesich. He was a senator at the time and it was our mother ship in Bristol Bay.

Aboard we had some Aleutian Eskimos and when I got home I had a wheezing in my

chest. I went to a Dr. Law and he said I had T.B. and would have to go to a sanitarium for

6 months. We were in his office on the 18th floor medical/dental building. The window in

his office was open and I said I would jump out. I could not leave my family for 6

months. So within the next week we made arrangements or me to go to Col River, our old

fish home, for six months alone. I had to take 14 big white pills every day and stay away

from people. I also had to come in once a month for a check up. I thanked God for

working a miracle on this body of mine. I was completely cured in 5 months.

The kids, Dan and Deb, loved the river. We had relations around us in boat houses and

they had their fun on the nice sandy beaches. But we had to go home when the season

was over on August 25th each year. The kids had to start school. So mom started going

with me in May and September each year. She loved it on the river. We moved off the

isle and that was a hard decision but we had no lights and had to chop wood and all and it

was just too hard.

We moved to Pillar Rock, a small town one mile from Brookfield. Brookfield had been

sold to Crown Zellerback a big logging outfit and they made a log dump out of the town.

For the next 25 years it was a busy truck logging town with no one left. The Gregets went

to Pillar rock too. I moved up on the mountain and we had a filthy house but we cleaned

it up and made a nice home. We had lights, a refrigerator and water. It had an oil stove

and all electric stuff. It was nice and we lived there for five seasons which means several

years. We finally moved because a few of the kids in town were Indians and kept

breaking into our house and stealing and doing damage to the place. One winter they tore

it up inside and just wreaked it all. We ended up renting a float house over in Woody Isle

again and lived there a few more years.

In the winter I did different kinds of jobs. Every winter I drove an oil truck. I did that for

five winters. I drove a cab for five winters too. In 1957 I went to work for Gene Fiedlers

Chevco as a new car get-ready man. I washed and cleaned the cars and undercoated them

for $1 a car. I made $400 a month, $100 a week clear. I cleaned up to five or eight cars a

day for the showroom floor. They had to be perfect and I did a good job. I learned a lot

about cars. So in 1960 I went into selling cars as a salesman. I did real well knowing a lot

of people and fishermen. I sold a lot of cars and had my own way of selling, the honest

way. I was a good salesman. That was why they called me honest Dom. That became my

nick name. For 28 years I sold cars in the winter time. I quit in the summer and fished

and then when winter would come again I would sell cars again. I was fishing from Oct.

25 – June 1. We had up to 12 salesmen at times and they came and went by the dozens.

Some had college educations as well as all kinds of others but most couldn't make it.

After a few years I was selling up to 20 cars a month. I won all kinds of prizes, money

and I got to really liking it. With fishing and selling cars I was going 12 months a year.

Back in 1953 we had moved across the street in a nice home. I paid $9,000 for it and we

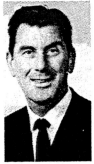

lived there for 27 years. I finally sold it to my daughter Debbie and when they sold it they

got $122,000 in 1991.

During the time I was selling cars there was this guy named Frank Novito. He and his

wife Helen were good friends of ours. He sold cars too and had done so for 42 years. He

was also a good salesman. We were already top salesmen and one of us was number one

each month. We had a lot of friends, there was Pete Blake, Don McDonald, Ed Keohara,

my neighbor Was Harry Stitz when we lived on 55th Street, and his wife Dorothy, they

were our friends for years. Harry died of a heart attack about 1986 or 87.

I could also write a book about my experiences as a car salesman. There were some

interesting things that happened over those 28 years in the winter time. The kids, Dan and

Deb, were all growing up and going to school. Nancy and Cathy were doing fine too.

Their family was taking care of them. We just kept on living. I was buying property. I

bought 43 acres of land in Vashion Island. I sold 20 acres at the present time. I have 14

acres and a farm with a small lake on it. It was a dream and I bought four lots in Ocean

Shores. I also bought four lots in Shelter Bay La Conner and sold them cheap. I had four

homes up until 1979-80 and I sold all the homes except my Vashion property and my

Ocean Shores lots. Deb and Dan were in high school and Dan was a real athlete. He

played football, baseball and basketball. He is tops in all the sports. Deb is a boys' dream.

She was pretty and has a nice boy across the street named Dale. He had his eyes on her

for a while. Things were going fine.

In1973 my mom died. I miss her very much. I was her baby and she was my mom.

Soon the kids were finally grown and out of high school. Dan had himself a nice yellow

truck and every winter we had a new car for 28 years. We had a demonstrator every year when I got back for the winter. We had a nice home and all the money we needed. Then

Debbie changed our lives forever. She ran away from home.

She was 18 years old and left with Dale, our neighbor boy. They left for Montana in the

middle of winter in an old Buick. It was a $50 car and they were going to drive it over the

mountains in heavy snow and ice. We were worried out of our wits until we heard from

them. I remember I wanted to beat my son-in-law to death at the time. I couldn't believe

it was happening. Mom was under a doctor's care and had to take pills to keep her stable.

We finally got them back to finish school. They lived in my rental house next door and

we helped them set up house keeping. They lived there while finishing school and of

course Debbie got pregnant right off the bat.

In the meantime Nancy and Cathy were going to college at Washington State. They were

going to be teachers and both got married and divorced. Both of them remarried. Nancy

married Rice Bahl a big husky Russian boy. They have one girl whose name is Karla and

two boys, identical twins named Leith and Jace. (I hope I spelled their names right) They

live happily on Whidbey Island. They have a home with a few acres and are doing okay.

Cathy married Tom Crownshield. He is an electronic specialist and they have three

children, one boy, Brice and two girls, Lindsey and Dreana. They live in Edmonds. They

have a nice home and are doing real well. I am very happy and proud of my family and

their successes. All my children are hardworking people as I always was.

My boy, Dan, became a truck driver and a tree topper. He is a work-aholic like his dad.

Dan married a nice girl named Betty and they bought five acres of land and a nice home

out in Maple Valley. He has two children; Kristine is a doll and papas girl. She has been

around me since she was a baby. I had her on Vashion wth me for days at a time and we kind of grew together. Then there's Joey, he's another Dan. Joe is a white haired little cutie. He is a nice and loving boy. His name was to be Dominick after papa but it turned out to be Joseph Dominick. He's a worker for a little guy.

Deb and Dale now have two boys, Dominick, named after me. He had a few problems and didn't want to listen to papa. I practically raised him. He was our 1st grandkid and we love him a lot. Sean, his brother was born next. He is a well built athlete type of kid. I hope he goes somewhere with it. I think he will really be somebody someday. Dale is a city bus driver and Deb is a receptionist for our baby doctor. They both work and are getting along.

It was at this point that the doctors discovered I had a tumor on my breast. It was growing fast and I had a biopsy. It was malignant and the doctor said that we would have to try some radiation. I told him, no cut it out and do it tomorrow. He went my way and everything turned out okay. I healed once again quickly and went off to start fishing on the Col River. It was the month of September.

Chapter 20
Cancer

This is how I first discovered I had cancer. On September 11th I went to the doctor, Dr.

Lading. He checked my prostrate and took a biopsy. He said I had some bad cancer

tumors on my prostrate. He suggested that I should have them operated on within the

week. My fishing season was about to open too on September 13th and I told the doctor

that the first week was only good for fishing and we would have to do it when I got back.

By the last week of September I left for the Columbia River fishing and it was a big fall. I

felt good and kept fishing up until the last of November.

I got home and the doctor set me up for surgery. I went into the West Seattle hospital.

After my surgery I woke up and felt real good. The doctor came in the next morning and

said I could go home but to come to his office in a couple of days. Two days later I had

an appointment with Dr. Laidig. My wife and I were ushered into his office and the doctor

sat us down. He said "Dom, Mr. and Mrs. Budnick, I have very sad news for you, we just

opened you up and sewed you right back up. You waited too long. I told you to come in

three months ago. Now the cancer has spread to your glands, muscles and prostrate.

You're full of cancer, "With tears in my eyes and I noticed his eyes watering up quite a bit,

I answered with what can be done. He said "Probably nothing Dom, I'm sorry. We will

have a talk with some other doctors though and have another look at your x=rays. My wife

wiped her eyes and I asked, "How long do I have Doc?" He said I was strong and would

go for five to six months at the most. I thanked him and went home to wait for the end.

The doctor called a few days later and said Dom I'm sorry but you better take care of

your business and family. He said he would be in touch. He also ordered 100 morphine

pills to cut my pain down.

I went to West Funeral Home and bought a whole funeral plan. I bought a casket. I even

took my shoes off and got in and tried it out. My wife ran out crying but I felt

comfortable. The little woman who showed me the casket said that this was the first time

in 20 years working there that she had ever see anyone do that. As far as I was concerned

that went well but it was at this point that the problems began.

With my funeral plans all done I had other things to do. In 1965 I had bought six plots in

Calvary Cemetery and two mausoleums. I had also bought my stone and a gold sealing

vault. When all this was ready I went up and saw Father Malahan from our church, Holy

Rosary and asked the church to pray for me. They also had a lot of other churches

praying for me too. He, the Father, came by my house one day a week. He walked one

mile from the church to my home and we said the rosary together. We talked, prayed and

had a cup of tea. He was a real good priest. Sometimes he would come three times a

week.

Time was passing and I was losing weight. I couldn't sleep at night. I would be sitting up

wondering what would become of my children. Dan was going on 30 years old and was a

very good boy. My brother Gus always told me that Dan was his son also. Gus really

loved Dan and my daughters. Debbie was 32 years old now and doing well. She's a real

mother hen, a nurse now. She also worked for Dr. Liagdig at one time and she was a real

fine woman. My other daughters, Nancy and Cathy were doing fine. They were all

married and had families of their own. I was hoping they could all go on without me.

I had some insurance but not too much so this was another worry. I was losing weight a little more and bleeding a little more. There was more pain. I prayed more and more.

There were problems with my wife Dolores. She and I had been married 35 years and now going on 36 she might lose me. She had a mother, Leona Sell, that was her married name, and she had altimzers. She'd been a good woman but she had been sick a year now and that was stressful. We had made many trips to Everett to help her. My wife had a sister whose name was Dwyla Dietrick but she wasn't much help. My wife had a lot of problems with her own family. She was now leaving me home alone while she was going to the nursing home her mother was in. She would be there all week and would come home on weekends, wash her clothes and take off again. It left me at home cooking, washing laundry and taking care of the whole house. I was dying and her mother lived for several more years after all this. There was a lot going on with me within those six months. I was very crabby and I was in pain. Having to care for myself and home made it harder. Things got worse and it didn't get better. My wife and I were drifting apart.

So my days were getting close and we had a very sad Christmas. We all tried to be happy and we all went through the motions. We all went down to my brother Mike and his family's home. We spent all Christmas Eve at my brother Gus' home and that was hard too. Most of them didn't know I had cancer. And those who did know didn't know I was terminal. It was a very hard night. I was in pain and kept to the kitchen and bathroom. My brother Gus knew when I went upstairs to lay down for a few minutes. He came in and we cried together. I was like his kid and he had raised me for so many years, in fact until he died. He said I was like his son and we shared our stories. As he left the room he told

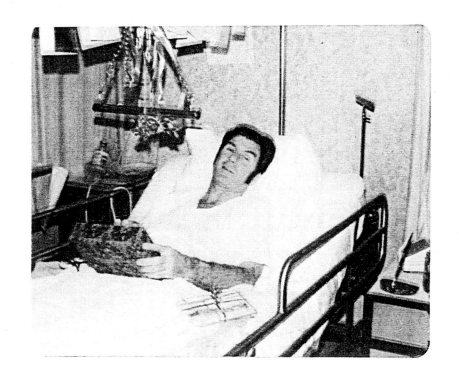

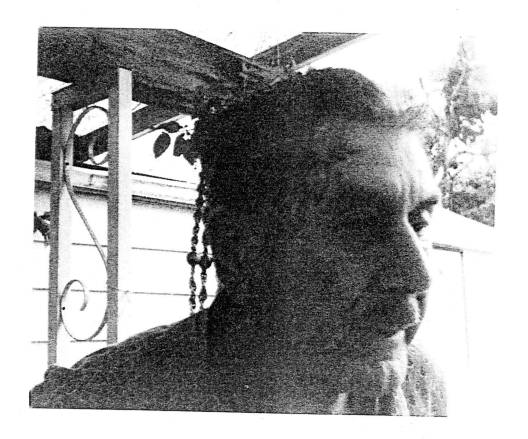

me, "Dom I am the oldest, I'm supposed to go first not you." He left and I never forgot those words.

Christmas passed and New Years came. I spent it lying on the couch. At 4 a.m., then 5 a.m., then 6 a.m. I lay watching the cars going by worrying and praying that I could go to work. I would cry myself to sleep. I wasn't eating much any more and I was using more pain pills, the morphine.

Dr. Lidgie called and said he would like to try chemo therapy. I decided that it couldn't hurt so I got to the hospital for the treatments. I take four shots of chemo and I get home feeling real weak and sick. My hair was falling out and my comb was full whenever I tried to use it. I called the doctors' nurse and said no more chemo shots. They didn't believe me when I told them I had gotten into my casket to try it on. I told them the next time I get in that thing I'm going in with a full head of hair. And I didn't go back for any more treatments. I had read somewhere anyway that chemo just prolonged life and it cost a lot of money. All my cousins died taking chemo.

So here I am waiting on the Lord for the day to come. The Father still visits me and I am going no where fast. I am in more pain then before, I have diarrhea and bleeding. The time is getting close. So days pass and there is no time for me. The days become minutes and nothing means anything. I am down to 120 lbs from 199 lbs. I fight and pray everyday more to the Blessed Virgin Mary. All my life if I wanted anything I could not get she got it for me. I was now asking for a miracle. I continue to wait.

Then one afternoon I woke up after being up most of the night praying and Dr. Liadie called and wanted me to come in. He said he had a deal for me.

Chapter 21
Another New Beginning

In 1980 I went down to Dr. Laidig's office he said, "Dom I have looked over your

records you have had two cancer surgeries, glands under your armpits removed in 1950,

you had a cancer tumor removed from your right breast in 1951. You had duodenal ulcers

in 1954 then you had TB in 1956 and spend six months and treatments and isolation. In

1984 we took a small cancer tumor off your prostate. Now I find you have a malignant

tumor on your left shoulder. That's pretty to touchy surgery. I have been talking to Dr.

Thompson about your condition. I've called you in because I have been talking with the

stomach doctor, a nerve doctor and another urologist and the four of us would like to go

in and see what we can do for you, if anything. But your weight is down; you are now at

121 pounds from your regular weight of 192. You have only several months left at the

most. We will go in and do all we can to save your life. He said we kind of need a

miracle and I said well I have enough churches and people praying for me.

He said we will need a lot of paperwork signed for their protection. We think you have a

10 percent chance being as we issue are. Now I'm telling you, he said, No. 1, you may

not come off the operating table alive. No. 2, he may have a lot your parts missing and

No. 3, you may have a lot of extra pieces like pig intestines in you. You may end up

disabled and some part of your body but if you make it you will at least be alive. So in a

few days I was back at the doctors' office to sign approximately 10 papers. I figured why

wait I am suffering with pain and my family is suffering also so let's go.

I went in and the priest gave me the last rights for the fifth time. I kissed my wife good-

bye and head for the butcher shop. That's what we call it back then. In the operating

room where nurses, for doctors who introduced themselves and told a few jokes. I went out cold and it was 8 ½ hours of surgery. They gave me 9 ½ units of blood. When the

surgery was over I was alive at least and I was breathing. I was put into intensive care.

My wife told me that the doctor told her that I didn't look good. My pulse was weak and

he told the nurse to call him and any time of the night if I died. He said to my wife it's up

to the Lord now.

I was an intensive care for seven days when I came to. I opened my eyes and my wife is

there. I try to move but could not, my legs were dead. I had no feeling in either leg. I

was rushed into scans and tests at once. My nerve doctor was there; his name was Doctor

Owen as well as Dr. Laidig. They told me they had to take everything out in my lower

part. They had to cut into my nervous system the cancer had spread to both muscles and

nerves. They did all they could to try and save my life. They cut out all they could and

they said I probably would not walk for at least two years may be more.

After 21 days in the hospital, (something I would never forget the rest of my life was the

day when the doctors and nurses came in and closed the curtains and started to take my

stitches out. I was watching TV and it was a big day because they were launching the

space shuttle Challenger. It was when the teacher was going up in space. So we were

watching as the doctor was taking my stitches out and God the thing blew up right as we

watched. We all cried as the doctor and nurses with shaking hands finished the job.

(That's a memory I will never forget.)

After I came home to recuperate from my $128,000 operation, thank God I had some

insurance to help pay most of the cost, I was alone. I could not walk and my kids came

when they could and helped. My wife was up in Everett taking care of her mother who

was in a home and didn't need help. That's where my troubles began. I decided one day

I had clothes to wash, so I got all my bags; I had a colostomy coming out of one side for

my stool in another bag on either side. I had tubes coming out all sides. There are 22

steps down to my basement and I started step-by-step backwards on my knees, bags and all.

I made it to the washing machine and reaching up I got my clothes and started the washing.

I started back up the steps and I noticed blood in my bags so I got the phone and called the

doctors office. The nurse answered it as I started to talk the phone cut off. Now I had no

phone and bleeding pretty good, I didn't know what to do so I crawled to my big front

window and there the city light crew was working on a pole outside. I banged on the

window with my cane and screamed and yelled but no one saw or heard me. After 15

minutes I got to the front door, crawled, bags and all, onto the porch and scream for help.

Finally the foreman of the crew outside heard me and I told him about the problem. He

called the doctors office on his cell phone and the doctors' nurse drove up to my house.

She took me to the hospital and there they found out I broke some stitches inside

somewhere. I had done so stretching in the basement so they opened me up and fixed me

and then sewed me back together again. In a few days I was home again.

At this point my life gets worse, I have troubles with my wife, and she's still going up to

her mother's. She has her own problems with her mother, my wife, but with my cancer

I'm very crabby and cranky and hard to live with. I was, or still am, a very active hard-

working man. It was hard to be in the shape I was and finally we realized our marriage

was not good. (I found out years later that my wife had started to get Alzheimer's disease

at about the same time.) So after five months of dragging around the house with bags

attached to me and checkups with the doctors they called me one morning to come in and

see them. So I went in and they finally took my bags off and my tubes out again in a hospital for three more days. I prayed day and night that all would work out. I was at 109 pounds when I came in the hospital now I was at 158 and gaining, so there was some good news. My plumbing was OK and I would not need more bags. I was put on a special diet and I had to eat baby foods for a few months but it was all working thanks to God. (And some good doctors)

After six months I was starting to walk by sheer willpower. I was exercising and forcing myself to move. My children I will tell you that if you have the willpower to have it all. I am in better shape now because of it. But I'm still alone.

I had this 10 acre land on Vashion Island and I had a 66 foot trailer and right below where my trailer sets there's a small lake with about 1000 trout in it. The geese come down in the spring and stop off and nest. The ducks come too. My family moved me to Vashion and put my bed and in the front room by the big window so I could watch the birds, deer and other animals while I recuperated. I would get out in the sun and sun bathe and for the rest of the summer I would get stronger and thank God I was alive at least for a while.

During my last visit to the doctor he said there's no guarantee and he gave me one to five years. He said that if I make that I may have a chance for more time so, he said, enjoy yourself, go and travel when you get better. Knowing I had maybe five years to live I decided to do what he said.

The summer was about over and winter was coming. My wife had a cousin who had a condo on the beach in Honolulu Hawaii so I call them in California and asked if I could use it for the winter. He said okay and I left for the winter in the first thing I did was bought a lot of writing paper and pens and they started writing my book.

My life was changing that I was doing so many new things in my old age. Have a friend

in Hawaii who owns or leases 25 acres of land and on this land he grows papayas and

bananas. I went to his farm in Ponalulu, its called Kapaka farms. His name is Bert

Pastana and he has a dad who was 70 years old also worked with us. Bert is a very hard-

working kid. He's the hardest worker I've seen in years. He never stops and he has a

helper whose name is Sepu. He's a big husky Samoan boy and he really knows the

papaya and banana fields. He knows what to do and how and when to pick the papayas.

He is a pretty nice guy he plays rugby football a real tough sport. So I went over every

Wednesday and caught a bus at 5:30 AM I travel two hours to get there. When I get there

I jumped in some clothes so old and dirty that the pants stand by themselves. The socks I

put on are as stiff as a board. There're black and dirty from being in the field. That is

what you need in the fields though.

We go out and start to pick the fruits. We use a toilet plunger. We attached that on to the

10 foot pole and we would go with the plunger and set it like a cup under the papaya and

push up and break the papaya loose. Then it would drop in and I would catch it and put in

a five gallon pail. When six pails are full we take them to awaiting tractor with boxes on

it and dump them into it and then do it all over again until we had about 50 cases. The

papayas are big; they weigh about 3 pounds a piece. There are six to eight in a case. After

we picked them we would take them to the packing house and we would sit at this bath

tub and cut the stems off and put them into fresh water to wash them off. After washing

we would pack them in boxes and weigh the cases. A papaya tree grows in one year and

the reason they are taken down or dug up at the end of five years is because they would grow too tall to reach the fruit. Papaya trees bear fruit all year long and it is amazingly good food for the stomach.

We would also do bananas. Banana trees are cut on to get the fruit. It takes a year for a tree to grow and then it is cut down when the large bunches of bananas are yellow. You slice the tree with one chop using a machete. You have to catch the tail of the bunch of bananas as the tree is falling. You pull on the tail and hold I up so the bananas don't hit the ground. There's a special knife that you cut the bananas with. You cut the bananas off their stems and back them in large banana boxes. The boxes weigh about 30 lbs and there are about 40 bananas per box. There are different kinds of bananas, the Chinese banana is red, but they are good eating. The best banana is the apple banana. There is also the Rey Tony banana and the icream banana.

We cut the banana tree about 3 feet from the ground and dig it up by the roots. We then replace it. We replant the whole field, it is very hard work. I planted 200 trees and I would get tired, but I enjoyed the summer. When summer came it was finally time to head back to Seattle.

I had spent 6 months in Honolulu and I had really enjoyed it. The sun and the swimming had done me well. But the wife was also there and she did not care much for it. So we finished my winter and sport fishing days in Hawaii and headed back home and all kinds of trouble.

When we got home Swedish Hospital had been trying to get a hold of me. They had been trying for several months. When I called they told me I had to take an AIDS test. I was told that 72 surgeries had been performed at the time I had had my big one and that there had been 11 cases of AIDS contracted from the blood used. I went right away and had my test and then headed for the ocean. I was gone 4 days when I got an emergency call from

my daughter Debbie who said I had to come home because my blood was bad. I rushed

home and boy what a time. I found out that I didn't, in fact, have AIDS but that my blood

was full of cancer cells.

At this point my wife announced that she wanted a divorce. We went and saw a lawyer at

once. We went through counseling at church but we finally gave up. We were just apart

too much. She hated Hawaii, Ocean Shores and Vashion Island, everything I liked she

hated. So we went our separate ways.

After the paperwork was finished for the divorce I went to the doctor and had further tests

done. I decided that while I waited for the results I would go to Vashion Island and take

my favorite grandchild, Kristine. We went for just a day or two and while we were there I

played with her a lot. One day I was tossing her into the air when I got a pretty good pain

in my lower stomach. I thought, oh no, I'm in trouble again. I left the island and went to

the doctor again. He said I had ruptured myself but that he could operate in a couple of

days. They operated and found a tumor down in my stomach that they had missed. I

ended up in cancer surgery again. This one wasn't as bad as some of the others though. I

went home from the hospital and was able to be by myself and my daughter Debbie

would stop by on her way to work to check on me. She also would go home after work;

they lived about a mile away, and fix dinner for her family and then come and take care

of me. She did this until I was healed. She is a very good daughter, my daughter Debbie. I love her very much. I will never forget everything she, as well as the rest of the family,

has done for me. I truly love them all.

Chapter 22
On My Own

Summer was finally over once again and I headed for Hawaii. I had decided not to go back to fishing on the sport boat but to find another job. So when I got there I got an apartment next to the beach and I swam and walked a lot enjoying myself for the first month I was there.

After the first month I got a job as a security guard for $5 and hour. My first job was in a million dollar condo building that had 20 condos within two huge buildings. As people drove into town from the airport they were on the left side and they were beautiful buildings. I had a big office and I sat and watched all the hallways, front doors and back doors on video cameras. It was a real neat job.

I spent the winter there and got back home to Seattle in April. I went in for my check up and here I went again. I was 200 lbs and I felt good and healthy but during my checkup they found cancer somewhere in my system so I ended up in the hospital again for tests. I was taking scans, x-rays and tests of all kinds. Finally they discovered I had tumors all through most of my organs. The doctor said once again that I didn't have much of a chance. He said they couldn't take all my organs out, I couldn't live without them. My daughter Debbie and I went through all the misery again. We left the doctors' office in tears and drove home. Once again they were saying I was terminal and all I had was 5-6 months. I went home and just stared out the window. I couldn't sleep and I was awake at al hours of the night. I just sat in my front room looking out the window wondering how much more suffering I would have to go through in my life. I wondered about the pain that was yet to come and worried about how bad it might be.

In the meantime my wife got her divorce, what she had wanted for the last four years, and moved to about two miles away from our home. She got an apartment on California Avenue and was living there. I was at home alone wishing as I looked out the window watching people go to work, wishing that I could go to work like them. It was a sad time in my life.

The doctor had said on my last visit to him that he would try anything he could but he still believed I was terminal. After that I stayed around the house, waiting, I guess, for the end to come. After one month of waiting I got a call from Providence Hospital asking if I wanted to come and talk with them about maybe possibly doing radiation treatments. So Debbie and I went to the doctor and talked with a Dr. Cole. The verdict was, if I wanted to, I could try a special kind of radiation treatment. I would have to have six shots at a time for a total of 42 treatments but it could burn my organs up and cut my time down to three months instead of six. They said it would be hard in the end and it might prolong my suffering and the suffering of my family but in the end we decided to go for it. Debbie and me cried again all the way home. It just isn't easy to give up life when the time comes.

I went to the hospital and got tattoos in six places. I was measured and after a week I was ready. I started with five days a week, two days rest and the others with radiation. Getting the radiation treatments was not bad at first. I had fun with the nurses and the Priest and nuns would be there every morning. They would counsel me before treatments. There was also a 1000 to 5000 piece puzzle on the table there to work on while you waited for your turn for treatment. The nuns and Father always had a joke for you and the counseling made you feel good.

Some of the sights I saw there were terrible and depressing. I met people and kids that were at the end. I knew people who would soon leave this earth for a better place. It was sad at times.

As far as the nurses go, we had fun. I told them in the beginning that I was going to Hawaii again for the winter and they all joked that they would be going with me. We joked about a lot of other funny things too but I was sure I was going back to paradise, as they called it.

Things got bad and then they got worse. I was bleeding, vomiting blood and I had diarrhea so bad that I was living in the bathroom fifteen hours out of twenty-four. I was hurting real bad. I didn't know that a body could take so much pain and suffering. I thought I had gone through hell before but at that point I really knew what hell was like. They gave me pills to help. I was taking Lomitil and Amodium pills, up to 10 or 12 a day but it didn't help. I was eating less now and losing weight again. I was ready to give up. We had my birthday party at Deb's yard and on that day I thought I was finally at the end. I bled so badly that I was surprised that there was that much blood inside a person. I went back to the hospital the next day and they told me they would have to stop at 35 treatments. They said I was all burned up inside from the radiation treatments. They filled me up with some kind of freezing foam, put it up inside of me, and sent me home. I did not have a bowel movement for weeks; there was nothing but blood and mucus coming out. But did grandpa give up, no way. I got Deb and we went to Costco grocery store and bought a bunch of food for me. I was going to force feed myself. I bought bread, big blocks of cheese, three jars of peanut butter and crackers. I put my table in the bathroom and my TV in the tub and sat there and forced myself to eat. Everything I ate would come back out, I would vomit or have diarrhea. I would make a big sandwich and eat one and it

would come back up. Sometimes the food would come up full of blood but I would just

eat another sandwich. I did this for 17 days and finally I had a small bowel movement. I

was so excited I called my doctor at Providence and told her. She wanted to see me again

so back to the hospital I went. I told her my story and they decided to try more radiation

treatments but I had to sign a special paper in case they should burn my organs out. It

said they were not libel.

So back I went and had 12 more treatments. I was going to finish this up one way or

another. My body completely changed during the last treatments. I was so weak I could

hardly drive or walk. My daughter Deb as well as Dan and his family came to the house

and all of them helped me. They helped all they could but it was hard on them all. They

wanted to do more but they had lives too. Being that I had been alone most of my life, I

knew how to take care of myself. I would just do the best I could. At that point in my life

I had already lost a few of my friends. Their problems were over but mine were yet to

come.

August came and I was on my last treatment. All during the last week they were probing

me and going inside my back end and taking scans and x-rays. Finally I had to go into the

office and visit with my doctor. I figured this was the end. I sat down and the doctor, she

had tears in her eyes, I knew I was done for. She finally said her tears were tears of joy

and tears of sorrow. The sorrow was because they had just lost a friend I had made while

I was there. He had died that day. The joy, however was that they thought they finally

had me in remission. She said I may actually come out of all this after a while.

She explained to me that all of my tumors were the size of grapes and there had been six

bunches in my organs and now they were burned down to the size of raisins. She said we

would know in one month if a miracle had been preformed.

I am writing this now in front of St. Augustine Church in Waikiki Hawaii with tears

streaming down my face just thinking about it all. How I left the doctors' office that day

and made it home with tears in my eyes and crying all the way to tell my children. I

called them and cried the whole time I told them and then I cried most of the night. You

don't go through what I went through and not cry with relief. I can not believe the

suffering and misery it was and worst of all, I kept thinking I wouldn't get to see my

grandkids grow up and all. Well, but here I am. I'm still breathing and working and living

a good life, a life that most people would like to have had.

I got ready to get my health back and gain my weight back. For the next few months I got

my strength back and when I was ready I packed and left for Hawaii. It was November 1,

1990. I had my old apartment which was not so good but it was okay. I came back to

paradise and got in the sun and began to build my body back up. Things were finally

okay again.

One day I went to Fisherman's Wharf and met some people there. I met a Captain Wally

Talbot and his mother. We got to talking and he said he needed a crewman. I explained

that I could do it. I told him about my commercial fishing experience and all my other

experiences all over the ocean and he took me on.

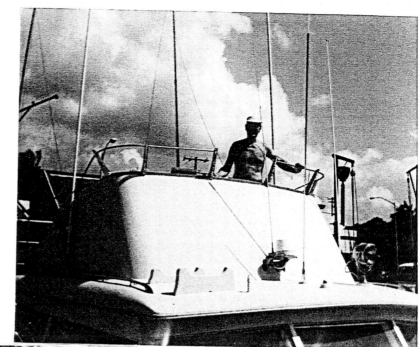

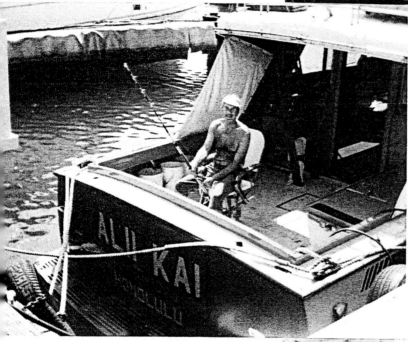

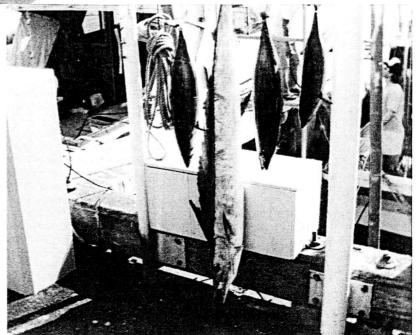

Chapter 23
Once Again

I ran and worked the sport boat the Ali Ki for the next six months. The winter passed

though and as sad as it was I had to leave another of my new adventures. Here I was on a

charter boat cruising the ocean and it was a beautiful life. We were fishing for marlin

swordfish, Mai Mai and tuna "Ochi Ochi". I left at 6 a.m. in the morning after I picked up

two 50 lb. sacks of ice and put it in our big fish box. We had a party of six people come

aboard. We all shook hands and got out to sea. I put out six big poles, $1000 reels and

$250 worth of lures and set them all up. They were numbered one through six. I would

then take a deck of cards and tell the six people to draw a card. The number they drew

was the number pole they would have. If the pole they got struck then the fish belonged

to the person who had that pole. That person had to pull the fish in. It is really exciting to

see a reel smoking out 1000 – 1200 feet and a marlin shooting out of the water on the

other end or running through a school of 5 – 6 miles of tuna. Or better yet, to see 100

whales all around you looking at you and jumping. It was a beautiful life at my age to be

able to see the sights I've seen out on the ocean. To see flying fishing sailing in the air or

porpoises by the hundreds, you just feel lucky to be alive and enjoying these things after

such a hard life. I worked the fishing boat for the first month.

I have done so many different jobs in so many different places. I have also done all kinds

of things in my old age as well. But it was time to head home once again to Seattle and

get ready to go to Ocean Shores. I had my check up and the doctors said they were

surprised that my blood count was okay. They said it looked like I would go on for a few

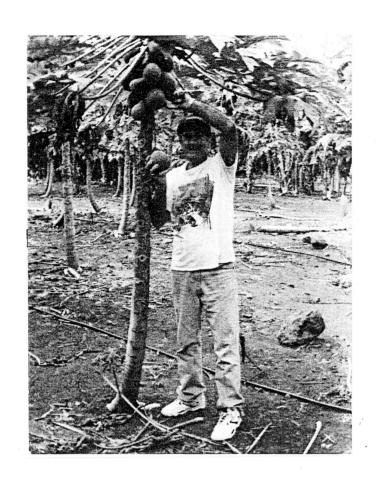

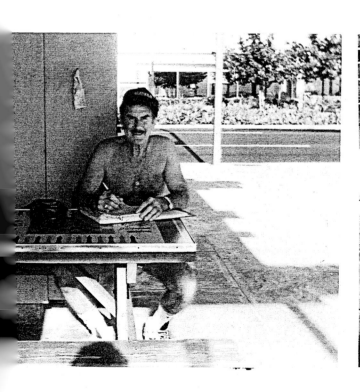

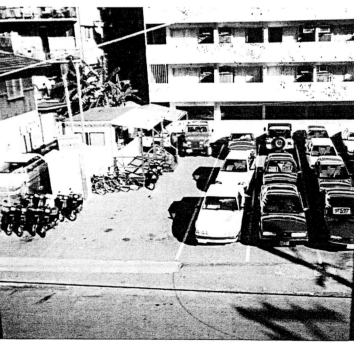

more years. So I headed for Ocean Shores. I work on a couple of lots I have there

sometimes during the summer months. I have a small trailer and I spent that summer

working on the lots. With the trailer I live in it is like living on one of my fishing boats. I

was a little cramped but I'm used to that.

The summer passed and I headed once again back to Seattle. It was moving into late fall

and one day while I was out I ran into my ex-wife on the street. She invited me to dinner

and we ended up spending the night together. She was lonesome so she moved back in

with me. She went with me to Hawaii and we got an apartment there, it was the same one

we stayed in before together. One month later I got a job right across the street from our

apartment at a car lot running a car rental agency. The people who owned it were Wilma

and Milland Wong, they were Chinese and really nice. I took over the whole lot of 60

cars and I rented them out as well as took them back in and collected the money for them.

I opened the place at 7 a.m. and closed at 6 p.m. six days a week. I had one day off and

an hour every day for lunch. When the bosses came in I would take off for the beach and

swim for an hour and they would bring me lunch every day. I liked the job. I made $5 per

hour straight time and that was it. I averaged $1200 a month for the time I put in but it

was tough. Sometimes a lot of people mean a lot of problems. It was not always a fun

job. I finished working the May 1st and I quit the job at Apollo Rent A Car. (The address

is 134 Uluniu Street in Honolulu, Hawaii, if you get to Hawaii kids stop by. Dad and/or

grandpa has a lot of friends in Hawaii now who liked me. They knew I worked hard)

We headed back to Seattle and of course I headed for Ocean Shores. I sold my 19 foot

trailer and bought a bigger trailer. (33 feet and nice.) I put it on our lot and started

working on both lots. I had the two lots cleared and had water and power put in. I thought

I had all I needed. I built a dock and it turned out real nice. It was for all the kids to use but with their jobs and all they very seldom came down. Ocean Shores is 2 ½ hours from Seattle but they had a hard time making it down.

I used my little truck and I went back and forth between Seattle and Ocean Shores. I would spend a week in Ocean Shores an then a couple of days at home and then back to the beach. I love the beach because I'm around water everyday. That is where I am happiest.

I finally went back to the doctor and took my regular physical. I was doing okay. I still had some bleeding problems and I had some more work done on my colon and the lower part of my body because I was pretty burned up from the radiation treatments. I have work done on it regularly.

So another summer passed by and the winter was coming and I was trying to decide what to do. I decided the best thing to do was to pack the trailer up and head for home where I would pack the house up for the winter and head into the sunshine of paradise.

On November 5th I get on a plane and head for Hawaii. I said good-bye to my family. I really do hate to leave them for the winter but my bones ache in the rain and cold of Washington winters. I have to go to the warm sun and try and put on a few more years to my life. I don't like to be away from my family though. I did try to get them to come to Hawaii and visit me. Deb and Dale came out and Sean and Nick and all of them were here in 89-90. I hope that someday my whole family would be able to go. It's a long trip but it is worth it.

I arrived in Hawaii and got a job right away with the Honolulu Police Association as a security guard. HPA was owned by a Hawaiian family and I worked the big hotel, The

Hawaiian Regent Hotel. That hotel had over 1000 rooms, it was one block long, it had

four bars, four restaurants, three parking lots, one tower that was 33 stories and another

with 25 stories, two tennis courts, two swimming pools and four ball rooms. It also had

meeting rooms. I got $7 per hour and all my meals free. They had milk, pop, all kinds of

pies , cakes, sweets and all of it was free. It was nice. I had a nice uniform, I got two sets

free, and the job was three minutes from the apartment. (If I walked fast)

I would work one eight hour shift, one 16 hour shift and two more eight hour shifts for a

total of 40 hours. I made $1104 in two weeks. One Christmas Day and New Year's Day I

worked 16 hour shifts. I got double time for those days because no one else wants to

work. I walked about three miles on a shift. I would patrol all the floors and the rest of

the time I would stand and listen to our music in the bar. I would patrol the elevators so

it's no work but I would meet a lot of people from all over the world. We had a few fights

and drunks that we would have to take care of. We had stores around our bottom floor.

One night a counter girl caught a man stealing and had him arrested. One time we caught

three people, all locals, peddling dope and we arrested them. It was a big bust, they had a

shotgun, pistol, dope and a lot of money in their room and we got them. They were all put

away from a long time.

It was an interesting job and my ex-wife came over for the month of Christmas and she

had a good time, stayed with me and all but she was on the go all the time so there was no

change there. She left after New Years and I found myself in paradise alone.

Chapter 24
Delores

The last week in Hawaii was beautiful that year. The weather was beautiful, in the 85

degree range, and the sea was like glass. The sunsets were out of this world. The sunrises

were just as pretty. The beauty in my island paradise took my breath away that year. It

was January 20, 1991 and the sea is like a mirror. I almost couldn't wait for sunset and

the moon rising in the clear skies. This was Hawaii at its best. I had had a beautiful winter

here working for the hotel. I had even been called into the office and given a special job

to catch and arrest the prostitutes in the area. There were a lot of them coming into the

hotel at that time. I was arresting up to 2-3 a day, 8-10 a week. On the street I was doing

too good a job and a few of the pimps got a hold of me. They wanted to pay me off but I

refused and the Samoans I worked for had run-ins with the pimps over me so I had to get

out of town real quick. I decided then to leave Hawaii for home.

Back in Seattle I didn't say much about my Hawaiian problems but I did get a check from

my boss plus a $500 bonus but I was also told not to come back to Honolulu for a couple

of years until things calmed down.

So I was at home and feeling good. Everything was calm. I went back to Ocean Shores

for a while. That summer I was having my coffee breaks in the sun and having fun with

my grandkids on the ocean.

Summer soon passed on the ocean though and I met some more nice people. I spent a lot

of time at the Community Club, our club we belong to, exercising and swimming. I also

spent time walking the beaches. That summer was one of the calmest I remember.

At the end of the summer we put the trailer away and headed home. Winter was coming and I couldn't go to Hawaii this year. So what was I going to do? Everyone in Ocean Shores heads for Arizona so I decided I would too. We flew down to Phoenix and we took a look around Mesa. (My ex-wife went along too) There were a few parks and finally we found a 70 foot 12 wide mobile home for sale. It was completely furnished and so I bought it. The trailer was all in my name, completely mine.

We flew back home and my ex-wife and I loaded up her new Buick and we headed south for the sun. We were now officially snowbirds.

We had a terrible trip down. We drove late at night and got lost down around Vegas. We finally found out we were about 40 miles from Vegas and headed for Utah. We ended up in a cheap rundown motel and had a really bad time.

Finally we made it to our new home and we had an adventurous first month. We traveled all over Arizona, saw the lakes, prisons and the Biosphere up in the mountains. I finally got bored though and had to find some work. I saw a help needed sign at a huge Kmart store and I got a job there. I was stocking shelves, being a security guard and a guard at the front door. My ex-wife was very unhappy that she was alone with a workaholic. I went back to work and that's when more trouble started.

My ex-wife was back at her same old routine, she had not changed a bit. She would get up at 6 a.m., go to the club and make coffee for the men; she would then have exercise classes, fist aerobics and then line dancing. Then she would stop and have coffee and then head to the big malls, have coffee again and then lunch and fashion shows. It was the same old routine.

I worked with young people and kept up with them. I worked more and harder then I had ever done before. The ex-wife said she wanted to live in Arizona but not me. I couldn't handle 110 degree weather, (and higher) in the summer. Heck it was hot enough for me in the winter there. I also loved my family, my grandkids and my kids. I was also lonely for my old gang. I always loved my family and my home. My heart even ached for them sometimes. I couldn't every live too far away from them. I guess I am just an old fashioned family man.

Christmas came that year and my brother Gus and his wife came down to visit us. They had a fair time. Delores was not very friendly to them and would not give up her routine. I took off work a few days to show them around but without a car though it was hard to show them around. Delores managed to cause a few bad deals there. She ruined Gus and Evelyn's vacation really. She was not nice and all crabby. If it wasn't about her she would change all at once. Gus and Evelyn finally left for home and everything went back to the same routine. All was going well when a few weeks later Delores put out the story that I had had a stroke and was in the hospital. Here I was working in the Kmart and the next thing I hear is that I've got a tumor in my head and I only have a short time to live. Delores made up the whole story. We all figured she must be on her way to Alzimers disease or something. We figured something was wrong with her.

For a while I worked eight hour shifts and she went on with her routine. She said I had my routine too and that I wouldn't change it for anyone either. She was continuing to get up at 5:30 a.m. and going to the club house making coffee for the men and then doing her exercise classes and line dancing. I worked to have something, that doesn't make me a workaholic.

The winter turned out nice despite Delores and at Christmas my grandkid Sean and a

friend came down and stayed with us for two weeks. They had quite a time. Sean and his

friend raised some hell but we didn't get kicked out of the park. We went up to the lakes,

Tortilla Flats and Tucson as well as Sedona. We went a lot of places. We had a real good

time at the end of 1992.

Going into 1993 the winter was a lot of work for me at Kmart. I loved working all my life

though and have done so all my life. My ex-wife said I was a workaholic every chance

she got. She said it, not once but 1000's of times in our marriage. She lived a good fancy

life though with fancy clothes and new cars and nice new homes with nice furniture and

lots of traveling all on my workaholic ways. I did it for 43 years but we were basically

happy in Arizona. But soon summer was coming and spring was already there so we

closed up the mobile home in Apache Jet and headed home. We went by way of Reno

and up to Portland. Delores's uncle and aunt who are real nice people lived there. We

spent a couple of days there and then took off for Seattle.

We got home fine. We took some time and got the house in Seattle all opened up. I left

for the ocean again though. I was beginning to like Ocean Shores more each year. I

would walk around the lots and have the same routine. I would hit the club for my two

hours of exercising and then have a good meal. I became a volunteer fire inspector and I

would go around to businesses and check their fire extinguishers as well as for fire

hazards. We would do this two or three times a week. That was a busy summer but it was

over quick. Winter was coming and so I closed up my ocean place and headed home

again.

That Fall we were getting excited about going to Arizona. We closed up the house in

Seattle and packed the car getting ready to leave. We stopped and visited Delores' Uncle

Francis and Aunt Iney on the way. This time we had a nice trip. We go there and started

setting up house. It was early October and we were early because most snowbirds don't

come own until the last of October. So we swam every day and went to the malls. We

met people at the club that was in the park where we lived. We traveled all over Arizona

and saw all the sights. The park is kind of for old people and I was getting bored. Delores

joined an exercise class and aerobics and goes from 7 a.m. – 11 a.m. I go looking for a

job. I went to Kmart and asked about a job. I was only going to work a few days a week

but I ended up working 40 hours a week, 5 days. It was a job no body wanted to work and

once again I am a hero for doing that kind of work. Delores is alone again at the park

though and starts going to the mall regularly. She is not happy with the way things have

worked out but the weather is nice so for a short time we were okay anyway.

The winter was going along fine that year and I was beginning to work 6 days a week.

Time was flying by and by February I had no idea anything bad was about to happen.

That year ended up being the worse one since the year my first wife died. It all started on

a Monday morning.

That Monday was just like any other day. I started out going to Phoenix with my friend

Charlie for a physical. Charlie was going to take me to the doctor, it was all planned. I

went to the doctor and while we were there I bought a big 5 lbs. box of chocolates for

Delores and I told Charlie I was going to take Delores out that night. It was Valentines

Day so he kept me a way all day.

We got back at 3 p.m. and Charlie dropped me off at my house. He would not come in and left at once. I walked into the house and found the house cleaned out. All the walls were bare, the bedrooms were cleaned out, and she took all her clothes and all of my stuff. The blankets, sheets, dishes, glasses, knives, forks, the vacuum broom, the dust pan, she took everything. I about had a heart attack. I could not believe that she was gone and she had done all this. We had been getting along just fine. I just couldn't figure out why this was happening.

I got the neighbors and they couldn't believe what she had done either. The park was in shock. It was the worst mistake she could have made in her life but I think she knows that now.

My daughter Debbie and son-in-law Dale came down to Arizona to help me. First we checked with all her friends and they had not seen her. We drove around trying to find her or at least to find out why she had left they way she had.

After a week of looking for her and not finding her we went to visit my friend Charlie and his family. Delores' car was there next door, all covered over in an empty lot. They would not let us in the house and they said my ex-wife could not see us because she had had a nervous breakdown and was in bed. They said she was under a doctor's care. They told us that she didn't want to have anything to do with any of us, that we were only memories. Surely the doctors had been right and she had Alzimers disease at that point. She wanted a new life so I said fine. I went over to our place and put the home up for sale. I sold it within a few days. We got on a plane and flew home.

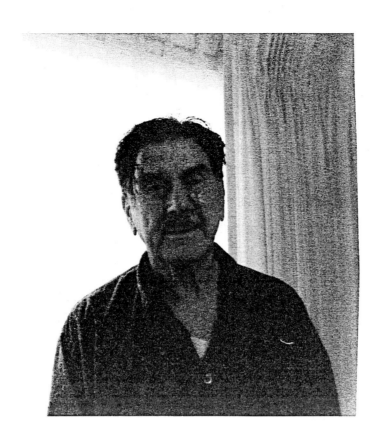

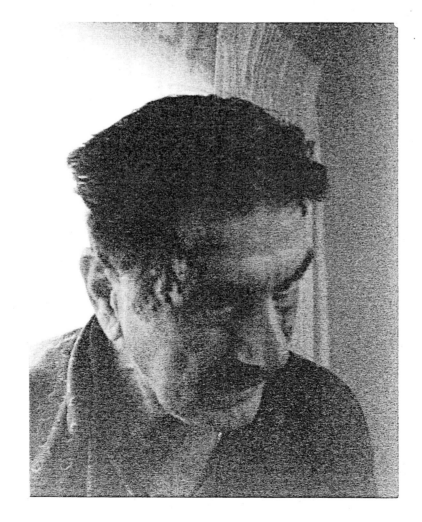

Chapter 25
Cancer Again

I went home and tried to settle in. What Delores had done had affected me a lot. I was

sitting in the house one day thinking about it all and I got a pain in the right side of the

top of my head. The pain was just at the hairline. I called the doctor and went in for a

check up. They did scans and tests and discovered that I had another tumor. They did a

biopsy right away and found it to be malignant. I think, oh boy I'm in trouble again but

then I think, maybe it won't be so bad this time.

I went into the hospital a few days later and they examined me some more. The first thing

the doctors said was let's do radiation or Chemo. I told them no you go in and cut it out if

you can operate. I wanted them to do it the next day if possible. I believe the only way to

beat cancer is to cut it out if you can.

I went into Providence and I had been there so many times that the nurses all run up to

me and say hey, Budnick is back! They ask what's wrong now and I tell them. The

started preparing me right away. The Father came in and we said a few prayers, then I

headed for the butcher shop.

This time they had to cut my skull open at the hairline. The dug the tumor out and then

closed me up. I understand they had a time sewing my scalp back together. The skin was

a little short so now I have some skin from my buttocks there. Now I know where the

saying comes from, "my face and your butt make a good match."

After a couple of days I'm back home and a little black and blue but they said they got

the cancer out. They said I should be clean now. I was at home recuperating and it was

1999. I had no idea that this year would turn out to be my worse as far as family deaths

goes.

Six months went by and I got a pain in my right eye in the left corner. They went in and

tested and found cancer. There was a small tumor on my right temple just on the inside of

my right eye. I had to undergo another biopsy and sure as my name is Dom it was

malignant. According to the doctors the tumor was the size of a BB but we watched it for

three weeks and it grew to the size of a pea. The doctor said it was growing fast so it had

to come out. This time I had to go to Highline Hospital out in the south for this one. My

doctor and my cancer doctor both wanted to work together on this one. Everything that

could go screwy will when it comes to me. The way they had to do the surgery, they had

to remove my eye out of the socket as far as it would go and tape it to the right side of my

nose. Then they would go in the hole at the right side of my eye but they ran into trouble.

They didn't figure that my eyeball was too big to get out of the eyelid so they had to cut

my eyelid in the middle and at the right corner. My eyelid had 22 stitches when they were

done and it wasn't a pretty sight. Everything else went well though and they removed the

tumor. I did okay for bout four months but then around March things went south again. It

started with my dad's brother in Portland. He had a sister, her married name was Berry

and she had a son named Gus Berry. He was my first cousin. He started the year off by

dying of cancer. This seemed to start a streak of deaths within our family. The second

death was Lisabeth Budnick in West Seattle and number three was William Budnick in

Portland. After he died his sister passed away too. Then my first cousin Mike Scrivanich,

my mother's sister's boy, died of cancer. A few months later Mike's sister Catherine died

of cancer and then the seventh to go was my cousin Larry Churlin. I dearly loved Larry,

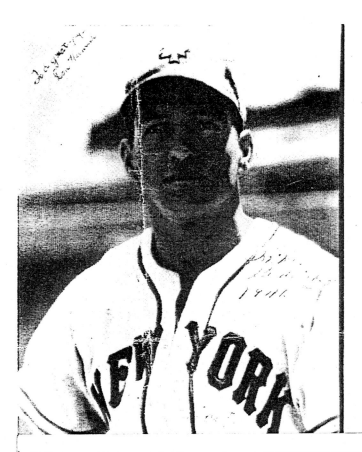

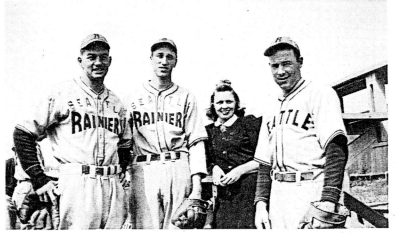

we were practically raised together. We were like brothers. He had had open heart

surgery and when complications set in he passed away. Number eight that year was my

brother Mike. He was a good strong ball player. He had pitched for the Seattle Rainers

and went on to the New York Giants and played ball. Kids you have to see his album

sometime. He was called Fireball Budnick.

Early in the Fall of 1999 Mike was diagnosed with bone cancer and was told he was

terminal. I spent a lot of time with him in his last few months. I helped him all I could.

He had goldfish out in his yard and he showed me how to water them with fresh water

twice a week and feed them. But he got weaker and was in more pain before long. He

finally ended up in the hospital in Ballard. It was Swedish Hospital and I spent the last

two weeks with him day and night. His wife Marge, she was a very nice lady, and I held

his hands for many hours until he finally passed away. I held his hand until he took his

last breath and closed his eyes. I gave him a hug and a kiss and left the hospital. His wife

and family left with me. Mike was 80 years old when he died, December 5, 1999.

I must have gone to a dozen funerals that year, most of them first cousins. There was also

my brother though and at the same time I had had three cancer surgeries at the same time,

all within six months. Not long after Mike passed my oldest brother was diagnosed with

cancer. In all I had lost 13 cousins and both my brothers within 18 months.

Before Gus found out that he had cancer he was having a hard time. He had a leg that had

retained so much fluid that it weighed about 50 lbs. He was in a lot of pain. He also was

taking my brother Mike's death pretty hard. He kind of gave up working and keeping

busy all the time and spent more time in the house. He was not feeling well most of the

time. He had had hip surgery and had a lot of pain there too. He had also had calcium removed on his back and was still in a lot of pain from that. Over the next few months he

spent a lot of time at the doctors' office doing scans and tests. He was finally diagnosed

with bone cancer which was the same thing my brother Mike had had. They told him that

he was terminal and so I spent a lot of time with him.

Gus had been both my dad and my brother. I would go down and visit him and he always

had a project he and I could do. We sawed a lot of logs and cut them up for winter wood.

We would pile it all in the shed. We also built a few chicken pens together, dug up his

garden and we planted vegetables. We worked well together. He was a very wise and

smart man, a good brother and dad.

Every time I visited him I would bring a special pastry that he liked. We would sit in the

kitchen and have a cup of tea and the pastry. Sometimes we would take a siesta for an

hour and then go out for our work he had lined up. One year we dug up his whole back

yard. He was trying to find the cover to his septic tank which was plugged up. It was

interesting to watch him figure that one out.

When he became house ridden he would signal me through the window telling me where

to dig. We finally found it and cleaned it out.

I always had fun fishing with him. We would fish off his dock. I built a break wind for

him too. I was in his shed one day and I saw some old lumber. I started sawing and

pounding and he yelled at me from the dock.

"What's going on up there? What are you pounding on?" He yelled. I loaded the deal on

his cart and brought it down to him. He couldn't believe it and we set it up and the wind

didn't bother him any more.

We loved each other down deep and from the time I was a young boy he treated me with

love and kindness. We had that old fashioned love for each other. (I am here in Ocean

Shores on our lot writing these few chapters and I have a lot of ducks here. There are

about five families of them with 10-12 ducklings. I'm feeding them bread all day and it is

bringing back a lot of memories of Gus and the ducks he use to feed.)

We use to go duck hunting and we had a lot of fun. There were a lot of exciting things

that happened to us to. We would talk about all our experiences quite often. I miss those

times.

Gus called me when he really started to get bad. He wanted me to come down to his

place. I headed down to see him and in the past we always took a drive once a day around

the island or up to the hatcheries up in the hills. This trip he was getting weak but he still

wanted me to help him up into my truck. He wanted to go to our old home town,

Brookfield. I knew by the way he acted and talked that this would be our last ride

together. He talked all the way down to Brookfield. He told me things I couldn't believe

and my heart was aching. I held my tears though. We got to where our old house had

stood on the hill and I opened the door for him. He cried and yelled. Why oh why he

cried. I cried too. By the things he said I knew he was close to the end. Despite the pain

we made it a nice day and when we got home we played cards every night. He was a

good pinochle player. We had fun every night, during the day we rode around the island

and he like this polka tape I had and always wanted to listen to it. I played it for him all

the time. After a few days I left for Seattle and then I finally cried. In fact I cried a few

times because I knew Gus' time was coming. I knew his time was short.

The following week I left Seattle for our place in Ocean Shores. I was going to spend

Saturday and Sunday there and then go on down to be with Gus again for the following

week. But on Sunday in the morning, Easter Sunday in fact, I got an emergency call, Gus

was in the hospital in Longview and he was in a coma.

I rushed down and the family was all already there. We all hugged and had our crying

period and then most of them left. I stayed for the first few days and nights with Gus. I

went home the following Thursday to get a change of clothes and head back but before I

could leave I got another call, Gus had died. My loving brother and father had passed

away that morning. I went back down for a few days later and spent several hours at the

funeral home with him. The next evening I closed the coffin for good.

The funeral was nice and we buried him on his 85th birthday, May 4, 2000. I stayed and

helped bury him then I put the flowers on his grave and left.

On Memorial Day I went to visit my brother at his grave. I visited him just like I use to

visit him at his home. I got a big cup of tea and the pastry he liked and a big bunch of

wild flowers and out it all on his grave. I played the polka tape he liked so much and sat

by his grave. I had a cup of tea and a pastry with him. I felt him there with me that day. I

stayed for an hour and then left. To this day I can't believe that both of my brothers are

gone.

Number ten that year was my cousin Lillian Tara Bochias husband Doc Sardrou past

away with cancer and that made eleven. Eleven in one year's time was almost more than

I could handle. I went to work at the church with the Father at Holy Rosary. The priests I

worked with could not believe how many I had lost in that year. With all the cancer problems I had you would think I would have been the first to go but I guess it's like

they say, the good die young first. If that's true I have a long time to live!

After my brother's funeral and all was done, I had another bad problem come up - I had a

pain in my left cheek below my left eye, pain I had for a couple months, I went to my family

doctor, he checked me out and sent me to my dermatologist, who looked and said we will

have to take a biopsy and let you know. A few days later I was called in and told I would

have to go see a specialist a Dr. Garegis. Here I go again! I was told that I had malignant

tumor (cancer) in my left cheek, so I was told we could try radiation treatments. I said no

thank you Dr., if I can have surgery that's what I want. He said it will not be easy I would

need plastic surgery and God knows what else. So as soon as I could get in to have the

surgery I went to Providence Hospital. The nurses and my priest was with me at all time,

they cut my cheek open in a V shape from the corner of my left eye down along my left side

of my nose on and 2 inches across and back up to the corner of my eye. It was a V up side

down. They peeled my skin back, went in and cut the cancer out. When I woke up in my

room, I looked in a mirror and looked like a real monster, I couldn't believe my face would

ever be the same again. It was terrible looking and did not feel good. The pain was bad for

a few days but again this was nothing new to me, all the cancer surgeries I have went

through, and may still go through. I feel very lucky that I am still alive, and again as I said

before and many times the word CANCER means put on the gloves and get ready to fight!

Chapter 26
Yet Still More Cancer

In March of 2002 I had another small surgery for a tumor that Dr. Watson at Providence

Hospital in west Seattle had found in the back of my head. He took a biopsy and there

was no cancer. He said it didn't look good though so he cut it out.

After that I got ready to go to Ocean Shores. It was April 5, 2002 and I was going to head

down there and get some rest and peace. It was clam digging season and I wanted to do

some crab fishing and get some sunshine. On April 7th I was in Ocean Shores and

volunteering for the fire department as a fire inspector again, I'm working out every day

at the club I belong to and I am walking two miles on the beach when the weather is nice.

When it isn't I can go to the club and use their machines. I feel pretty good. (I have been

writing this book since 1990 and people keep asking me where my book is. I had better

end this book real soon.)

I am keeping busy. I have some friends and they are on vacation so I am going to cut

their lawn as well as my own. It's been pretty hot this year in Ocean Shores. I am

spending my time here working on my book and it is bringing a lot of old stories to mind

like the time when we were fishing for the big cannery called Squaw Creek. The cannery

was owned by a big company called the A & P grocery chain. The company had a lot of

millionaire owners who had come that year from New York on vacation. They had heard

about the fishing. This one millionaire and his wife as well as three others flew in on a six

passenger plane. They had a private pilot and he stayed with us at the cannery for a few

days, When they got ready to leave it was a nice morning for flying. Some of the guys and I were watching from the bunkhouse as they took off. They went straight up about 300-400 feet and then started straight down to the ground. The plane hit and exploded into flames. What an awful sight that was. All those aboard were killed and it was in the New York papers. They called it a great disaster and a huge loss.

There was also one time when there was a huge storm. I fished for the cannery in the Nakneck River and we had six men with us all big oil company people. They were all going out on open fishing boats and we were going to fish on a 32 foot fishing boat. They were to drill in the shallow waters no matter what they had to do. A message was given to us that there was a bad storm headed our way. The oil men from different parts of the United States, with families at home waiting for them didn't listen to the warning or any of us old fishermen. They went out to do their job and the storm hit with 70 mile per hour winds and real rough seas. The men from the oil company didn't come back when the storm was over. After the storm 2500 fishing boats went out fishing and I heard that only four bodies had been found. We picked up one body, my cousins had found it but being superstitious they would not take the body aboard. I picked up the body and took it into our cannery. The body was wrapped in canvas and put under ice out on the dock. They covered the body with ice until the U.S. Marshall could come from Anchorage to pick it up. That was just the way of the wild north. Many lives were lost in Bristol Bay too. In past years there was a bank along the river where we fished. The bank is 100 feet high and it is called The Grave Yard. When storms hit against the bank there are coffins that stick out of the bank and bones have been seen hanging out of the bank. There were also bones on the beach below. It had been a grave yard in the late 1890's and early 1900's.

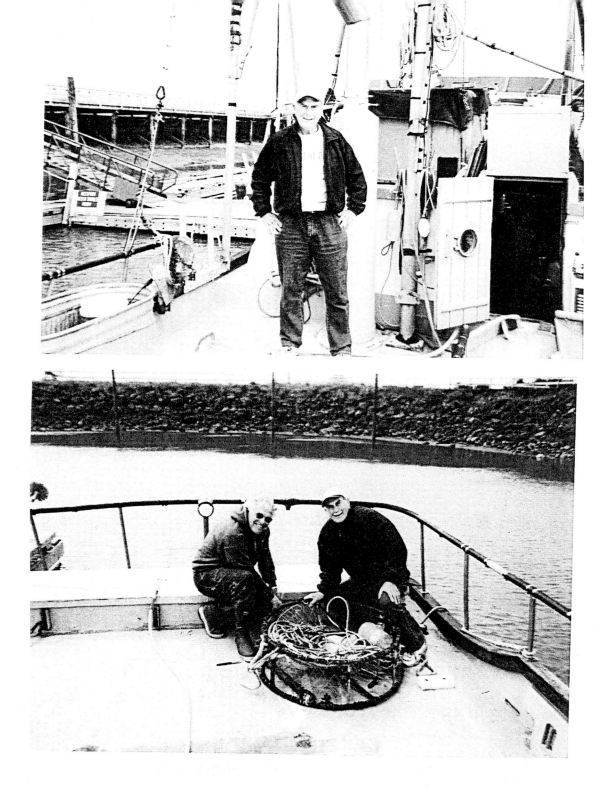
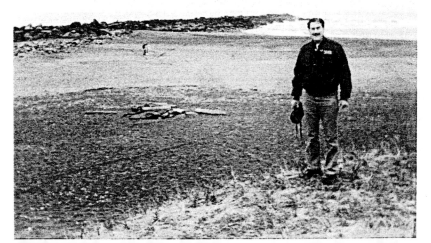

There were a lot of fisherman drown in the old sailboats in those days. Many of those

who died were buried there.

In 1950 the laws were changed and power boats were used mostly to save lives.

Note:

Life is not a big party or all fun and play. It is all hard work and trying to exist. You can

ask me, do not depend or wait for the golden years. There are no golden years: it is all

tougher, harder and full of a lot of suffering and pain. I am now 81 years old and what I

want to do I can't. I can't do all of the things I had planned to do in my 40's and 50's. I

am trying to do some of them now but even though the mind is willing, the body is weak. I

do go to the gym at our club in Ocean Shores and I walk on the walker two miles every

day. People who talk to me can't believe my age and my body. Most people guess me at

62-68 years old. I feel okay and good when I hear that.

There's a lot of new problems in Ocean Shores so many new rules and regulations,

ordinances and politics. After 43 years of enjoying it down here claming, fishing and

crabbing as well as much more I am forced to sell the property. We have had these lots

for years and I will miss it but I will have to leave the ocean for good soon. It was good to

be here for an old man, to rest and enjoy a few more summers.

I got notice from my doctor who had just examined me a few days earlier that I needed to

go and see my cancer doctor at Swedish Hospital. I went to see him, Dr. Green, he's a

very good doctor, and he said my PSA is very high and in my testicles. I asked what

now, and he explained that cancer goes from the prostate, which I no longer have, to the

testicles where your hormones sends it to other parts of your body. He said that was

why so many people die. They die because they don't try and stop it until its too late. He said we would have to do something soon. I spoke up and said how about

tomorrow. I told him to cut it out if it would save my life again. He laughed and said,

"Dom not so fast, we have to get an okay for an operating room and you have to have a

few days to prepare." I said I am ready, let's go. He laughed again and said go home and

we will make an appointment soon and call you. A couple of days later I was ready and

on the third day I went in to Providence. The nurses saw me and all welcomed me as

usual. The Father came to my bed and said blessings. He said Dom I have given you your

last rights and blessings so many times that I am running out of oil. I headed into surgery

again this time for the 12th time.

I woke up in the hospital and found out that all had gone well. I had another day, week,

month or year to live. The doctor came in and said they had cut my testicles out, scraped

them out and cut everything out around them, in other words they had castrated me. I

spent several days in the hospital. When I got home I couldn't do anything for two weeks.

Father Malhan came to the house and we talked for a while. I asked him, "Father how

come I am still here and my family, my brothers and my mom are all gone? I was told by

the doctors that I should not even be here after the 1985 surgery. With that and twelve

other cancer surgeries, why am I still here?"

The Father said, "Well Dom you are here because you are a giver and helper. You are

here to take care of your family and the girls and your boy. You have grandkids and great

grandkids to take care of."

I think I told the Father about 14-15 of them and I told him I loved and took care of them

all. The Father said, "The Lord sees what you have done and are doing and that's why you are here and will be for a many more years. Its hope and will power and prayers that

keep you going, just keep on doing what you have been doing in the past."

The Father left and I thought about what he had said. I think he might be right. I sat there

thinking about my past and I am doing pretty god now. I have been for many months.

I got a letter from my doctor a short time later and they wanted to see me and check me

out. They also wanted me to answer a bunch of questions so they made a 10 a.m.

appointment for me at the hospital. I called and said I would be in. I got there at 9:45 a.m.

and when I walked in the doctors were looking at my x-rays up on one of those lighted

windows. The doctor came over to me and said you were not supposed to be here. I told

him I had an appointment at 10 a.m. and he laughed and said that they had just been

looking at all my x-rays. He told me that I had had enough cancer in me to kill me over

and over again a dozen times. He introduced me to the other doctors and they gave me

sheets of papers with over 100 questions to answer. I answered them and then I was told

to undress and given a gown. They took more x-rays on several different machines and

they talked among themselves. They told me after four hours to get dressed. When I was

done the doctor came to me and said, "You are a very strong man with good will power."

He gave me a check for $50 and I signed it over to the Hutchinson Cancer Fund. I have

belonged to them for years. I always try and donate what I can to the fund.

The doctors took blood, urine tests and all and told me I'd get the results in a few days.

I am lucky to be alive. When I was fishing in Bristol Bay Alaska there were four times

when I should have drown. Several times fishermen right next to me drown. I can't, to

this day, figure out how I have gotten out of some of the terrible times I came through safe and alive. People, you have to have friends and you have to have will power and

hope. You have to have hope and prayer, here is an example,

Two friends went up to their mountain cabin. They got there and one says to the other I

will get a fire going and you get the small gun out and see if you can get a rabbit or a

grouse. I hope you get some food for dinner. He takes off out into the woods and he kept

saying I hope I can find our dinner out here. After hunting for a while he walks over a

mound and there is a big black bear. First he turns and starts running for the cabin

hoping all the time that the bear didn't see him. But he turns around and the bear was

coming after him. He ran and said I hope I get to the cabin but he got so tired he fell to

his knees praying, I hope the bear will not kill me and eat me. Soon he noticed that every

thing was quiet and he turned around and there was the bear on his knees. He looked at

the bear with his paws in the prayer position and the bear looks up at the man and says,

"hey young man don't get your hopes up, I'm just saying grace."

Chapter 27
Sacrifices

I was one of the top car salesmen at Gene Fiedlers Chevrolet for 28 winters. I cooked for

2000 people for the Hydro Boat Races at Seward Park for 2 years for Texaco for free. I

ran a 60 car lot in Hawaii for one winter at $5 per hour renting out cars and Honda bikes.

(It was a tough job) I washed cars for a rental company for $5 per hour and did up to 20

cars a day; I cleaned them inside and out.

I was a security guard for condos in Hawaii. They were 1 million dollar condos and

beautiful. As you come in from the airport they are the two big dark grey condos.

I picked and worked papaya farms and banana farms in Hawaii. (It was very interesting)

I fished for 62 years all over, in the Columbia River, Puget Sound, Alaska and all over

the ocean. I was a salmon fisherman, a gill netter, a purse seiner, a beam troller and a

bottom fisher. On all of these jobs I was called to come back and even today at my age

I'll bet I could go back to any of these jobs and they would hire me again. I have a very

good rating (100 percent) and a good reputation on all the jobs I have done. I am very

proud of my work record.

Now I could go on for hours about how I have saved and what and how I gave up for my

family. Saving as I have, I have always felt really good about giving and helping. I would

ask my kids to try giving. It will make you feel good.

Always do your job and do it well. Work hard at every job you have. My ex-wife Delores

was famous for asking, why do you have to be number one at every job you do? I was

number one and I am proud of it.

I was born to be a fisherman and I fished all my life but I also did many other jobs. I was a cookie baker in a cookie factory. I was an egg box maker. I worked in cold storage on turkeys and chickens freezing you-know-what off. I was a longshoreman for five winters. I was a cab driver for Grey Top Cab Company for two years and for Yellow Cab Company for three more years. I drove a fuel truck for Cascade Fuel Company for five years and I even worked for Harry the Kid Mathews Championship Fighter for a year. I was a partner in an Oil heating sales company for three years and had stock in oil. I was a gas station attendant at Richfield Station on the West Seattle Bridge. (The old Bridge) That was a cold winter and I made $1 an hour and worked from 12 noon until 8 p.m. It was a tough job too. I was lead maker at Pacific Marine. I made netted gill net and it took me a year to make it. I was the number one salvage net maker. I hung nets and was number one on speed. I was a mail delivery man. I was a parcel post delivery man for three winters for the United States Mail Service. I was a sport boat captain in Hawaii for two years. The best winter job I ever had was a security guard for five winters at the Hawaiian Regent Hotel. That was a good job. I was a feeder in a big fish cannery for one year and made $100 a month. I was a fertilizer sacker in a Port Ashton Herring Plant in Alaska when I was 14 years old. I worked for two winters at Kmart in Arizona as a stocker and security guard. I was a stocker at Payless Drugs for two winters in West Seattle. I was a tuna fisherman in the Galapagos Islands and Mexico for one winter. I fished sardines in the roaring twenties in San Francisco and San Pedro, California. I was a cook at a greasy spoon restaurant in Port Angeles for $1 per hour. I worked different jobs at the pulp mill in Port Angles, I made $1 per hour as a carpenter's helper for one winter in Fort Lawton. I made $18 a month cleaning and polishing new cars for one year.

I made $100 per month waxing and buffing cars for a body shop in 1959. I made $100 doing the same for Gene Fiedler.

Now my children, friends and all, you have read my book up to this point and I would like to tell you that it took a lot of saving in order to help you all. The great Depression of 1929-32 taught me how to save and keep from starving. I lived off of the city dump and you would all die of starvation before you would have done that. Here are a few examples of what it has taken:

My grandma died at the age of 79 and she had every tooth in her head. She had never even been to a dentist in her life. What I learned from her was not to use toothpaste. I have never bought a tube of toothpaste. I use salt. My grandma used a face towel. She wet it down and put salt on it and brushed her teeth. She never had a tooth brush. I use salt which has iodine in it and is good for the gums and teeth too. I have had very little dentist work done. I've cracked a few teeth by chewing on bones, which is good for strong roots and you also get every piece of meat off the bone like chicken. I have seen my kids and grandkids take one or two bites out of a meal or piece of chicken and leave it. I used to watch my mom clean up and eat the kids leftovers and I learned to not leave leftovers. I was taught to have clean dishwater when the dishes are done. I licked my plate many times when I went to bed hungry.

I make two bottles of soap out of one bottle of liquid soap. For years I've bought clothes from St. Vincent DePaul's, Goodwill and thrift stores. I have save thousands of dollars by making three meals out of what you all would eat for one meal. I've got closets full of good clothes and half are from family and friends who have died. I have lived on grocery sales, food sales and I have shopped store sales and saved hundreds of dollars. I also

bought the cheapest. It's always the same product just cheaper.

Listen to my advice and it may help. I have made many sacrifices for my family and I

hope that you all know how much I love you. I love you enough to sacrifice a lot.

Chapter 28
Leftover Memories

I was heading back to Seattle not long ago and it made me think about things. I will finish

my time on this earth in Seattle. I have a few regrets left over from my hard life. One

regret has to do with my first wife. My first wife never got out of the City of Seattle. All

she had wanted before she died was to see California. She had wanted to go south on a

trip but I never had the chance to take her. I didn't have the money at the time and I had

to work to be able to support the kids. It was too late too soon. When I went to the doctor

and asked if I could take her he said no. Even today I feel real bad and sorry that I did not

do more.

Another regret I have has to do with my mom. She could never read and write but she

was a very wise woman. She wanted to go places too. She wanted to go to California or

just to the ocean, Seaside, anywhere for a trip but with my own family and all I just

couldn't seem to find the time. I wanted to spend more time with my mom but now I feel

in my heart that I could have taken her on trips with my family. I could have spent more

time with her. But instead I have a pain in my heart and I spend a lot of nights going to

bed thinking of my mom and how much more I could have done for her. I think about

how many more days I could have spent with her. So do yourselves a favor and spent

time with those you love. Time is all gone before you know it.

This is not a regret but I figured I'd end this chapter with a funny story. I had a cousin

whose name was the same as mine, Dominick Joseph Budnick. In the late 1980's my

cousin died and his obituary was in the local newspaper. I was selling cars at the time and

I was pretty well known so when people saw the name in the newspaper they assumed

that it was me. It ended up being a real mess. We got cards and flowers from people and

they were telling my wife at the time how sorry they were that I had died. She even got a

letter from the teamsters union telling her when a check would come. It was a mess and it

took me some time to clear it all up. So you see I guess for some people I kind of have

already passed on. I'll bet there might still be some people out there who are shocked that

I am alive after reading that.

Chapter 29
In Closing

When people hear the word cancer, which is really no different than words like appendix

or ulcer etc., it's a word that means it is time to fight for your life. One thing it does not

mean is that you should give up. A good example is my cousin Catherine Scrivanich. Her

brother and many more I worked with handled things different.

One day I went by Catherine's house and she was home cleaning and had soup cooking

and she looked like one of the healthiest people I knew. Her brother Mike had passed

away one month before and so she was going in for an exam a few days later. I stopped

by after she had gone to the doctor and she was all slumped over in her big chair. I said,

what's up and she looked up at me and in a slow wavering voice and tears in her eyes she

said I've got cancer. I boomed out, "so what I've got a little cold, I've had cancer too,

how can you sit there when just two days ago you were running around the house like a

bee?" I told her that just because she was told she had cancer she didn't have to give up. I

told her to get up and keep working, I told her to move it. "You have to fight," I said.

"You have a fight on your hands look at me. You know how many times I have heard the

word cancer. How many times they have told me I have it? It doesn't bother me at all so

get up again." She said, "Why I've got cancer." She gave up right then and there. She

gave up at the doctors' office when she heard that word…cancer. She gave up and she

never got up from that chair of hers. Several months later she was gone. Several of my

friends and relations were diagnosed with cancer and I've gotten them up and moving and doing things but when I left them alone they would go back to the couch and finally

they too would leave this earth.

Since the death of my two brothers I figure I am next. I hope I am since I am now the last

of them and the oldest in the family. I am ready I guess. I've done all the damage I could

do on this earth and I only hope they, (up in heaven) don't laugh too hard. After all the

suffering I've gone through there has to be a heaven for me. I only hope they are ready

for someone like me. I am a religious person and have been all my life. I pray all the time

for my family and friends and I have helped a lot of people in my life. I have been ready

and willing for whenever and whatever to give and help. I have tried to be very generous

with my family, my children and everyone else. I only hope and pray that my family

comes out to my place of rest and visits with me. I know they say the spirit leaves the

body when you're gone but I believe that I will be with my family always. I've gone and

visited May on Christmas, Easter and Memorial day as well as many other times.

The ice cream I bought for years at 99 cents a half gallon that you buy for $4-$5 is the

right junk food. Other junk food like chips, salsa and other junk you never see in my

freezer or refrigerator because I remember. My lunches were not like the lunches you had

for school. I had two slices of bread with sliced onions and I ate that hiding behind the

school house so no one would see. Being poor was part of why I left and went to Alaska.

I am very much afraid of what the future holds for my grandkids. I will be gone by then

and not have to see it but at 81 years old I can see what is coming and it looks bad. There

are too many different mixes of the races and it looks like one day you all will be taking

pills instead of eating food. I think the day will come when there will be no more farms, cows, sheep and chickens. Some day all of it will be no more. Save ad keep your gardens.

Save everything you can.

As my mother and dad and my uncles lay every year up in the old cemeteries in Astoria,

Oregon up in the hills so I will go too.

I only hope that all my family and friends love me and respect me as much as I do all of

you. I am going to have a few copies of this book published so that you can read it every

so often. If you have any problems or sickness read my book and you will feel better.

Never give up the fight, use your will power and do a lot of praying. I believe the times I

have had terminal cancer I had a dozen churches praying for me. That is thousands of

people and right now I have, on my refrigerator, my obituary. It was in the P.I. a few

years back only it was actually my cousin. I guess next time it really will be me.

Friends many times I went into the hospital for cancer surgeries and I would be joking

with the nurses and doctors. I really had fun and I even remember telling a joke to the

doctors while I was on the operating table just before they put me to sleep. I am closing

my book now a last word of wisdom from a young 81 year old man.

When you hear the word cancer its time to fight and change that word from the word

cancer to the word healthy. Just do what your doctor tells you and keep living your life.

The life you were living before you got sick. Never give up. Just keep fighting.

I close this book now with luck and prayers, exercise and will power. In order to live, just

keep on living and loving. Help others and also be kind to everyone you meet.

Good health to you all.

Love,

Dom

My book is at the end now and is through, but as for me and my future life fighting cancer I am

afraid it is not. I will probably have more surgeries, MRI's, X-ray's, scans and meet more

doctors before my life ends. There will be an end though, with no more sickness but as for now

I will add a post script.

August 21, 2002, I have just had an MRI plus X-ray scan's and they have found out that I

have a growth on the bottom of my Vertebrae's. I was to be operated on September 28th

but due to the finding on my x-ray's and MRI I have some problems on my upper body, in

my face area. They sent them to my Dermatologist, Dr. Kulin. She took some biopsies of

the tumor's on my face, on my right cheek and found Malignant cancer under my left eye,

and on my left cheek. December 5, 2002 Dr. Kulin operated got what she could get out

and I was told by Dr. Kulin that the cancer on my left cheek and under my eye would have

to be operated on by a specialist, a Dr. Peter Odland, whom I went to see. He evaluated the

cancer and said I had to be operated on soon but I did not want my face all cut up like I had

several years ago. Christmas was coming so we made my appointments for the first surgery

under my left eye, January 30, 2003, then one on the cheek for February 23, 2003. My

lower back surgery will come after this book is published.

ISBN 1553954125-2